# Ejaculation Mastery: 10 Easy-to-Follow Strategies for Delaying Climax and Lasting Longer in Bed

## By

## Patti W. Nieves

**Disclaimer:**
The information provided in this book is for educational and informational purposes only and is not intended as a substitute for professional medical advice, diagnosis, or treatment. Always seek the advice of your physician or other qualified health provider with any questions you may have regarding a medical condition. The author and publisher disclaim any liability for the decisions you make based on the information provided in this book.

## About The Author:

Patti W. Nieves is a seasoned content creator specializing in sexual well-being, satisfaction, and pleasure for both men and women. With a passion for promoting healthy and fulfilling intimate relationships, Patti has dedicated her career to researching and writing about various aspects of sexual health and wellness.

As an experienced writer, Patti has a knack for translating complex topics into accessible and engaging content that resonates with readers. Her work aims to empower individuals to explore and understand their bodies, desires, and relationships in a positive and informed manner.

With a commitment to inclusivity and diversity, Patti strives to address a wide range of topics related to sexual health and pleasure, ensuring that her content is relevant and relatable to people of all backgrounds and identities.

Through her writing, Patti aims to break down stigmas and misconceptions surrounding sexuality, providing readers with accurate information, practical advice, and inspiring insights to enhance their sexual experiences and overall well-being.

Table of Contents

## Introduction:

Here you will learn how to master ejaculation, which is the art of slowing climax and making pleasure last longer in the bedroom. Let's start a journey of transformation through ten simple methods that will change the way you experience sexuality.

Think about this: You and your partner are in a heated hug, enjoying every moment of closeness without worrying about when it will end. Imagine being able to stay in a state of happiness and dance on the edge of the peak for as long as you want, all while getting closer to your partner.

But let's talk about why this journey is important before we get into the plans. Controlling your ejaculation isn't just about making sex last longer; it's also about making the private times better. It's about taking back control of your pleasure, letting go of time's limits, and opening up a world of physical options.

### Importance of Ejaculatory Control in Sexual Satisfaction and Relationships

Imagine a symphony, where every note is perfectly timed and harmonized, making a beauty of sound. Similarly, in the world of sexual happiness and relationships, ejaculatory control plays the role of the director, arranging the rhythm and strength of pleasure.

At its core, ejaculatory control is about learning the art of timing – knowing when to speed and when to stop, when to crescendo and when to linger. It's the difference between a fleeting moment of pleasure and a full, euphoric experience that leaves both lovers breathless and satisfied.

In the world of relationships, ejaculatory control holds the key to greater intimacy and connection. When partners can synchronize their rhythms, talking through touch and feeling, they form a tie that transcends the physical. It's about mutual knowledge, trust, and the shared goal of pleasure.

But the value of ejaculatory control goes beyond the bedroom. It affects our confidence, self-esteem, and general well-being. For many individuals, the failure to control ejaculation can lead to feelings of inadequacy, frustration, and even worry, impacting their relationships and quality of life.

By mastering ejaculatory control, we regain power over our bodies and our pleasure. We learn to listen to our wants, to respect the nuances of sensation, and to express our needs freely and honestly with our partners. In doing so, we develop a sense of empowerment and liberty that permeates every part of our lives.

Ultimately, ejaculatory control is not just about prolonged pleasure; it's about improving the entire experience of closeness. It's about savoring each moment, discovering the depths of sensation, and embracing the deep link that comes from sharing ourselves fully with another.

In this trip towards mastering ejaculatory control, you'll discover that it's not just about delaying climax, but about enjoying the entirety of the sexual experience. It's about learning to tune into the tiny cues of your body and your partner's, managing the ebbs and flows of desire with grace and confidence.

By improving your ability to control ejaculation, you'll open the door to a variety of options within your relationship. You'll make room for greater connection, more meaningful closeness, and a level of trust that transcends words. Each moment spent discovering your pleasure together becomes a testament to your commitment to mutual satisfaction and happiness.

As you gain control over your sexual reactions, you'll find that you approach life with a newfound sense of confidence and ease. You'll handle challenges with greater resilience, develop healthier habits, and foster more important bonds with those around you.

So, as you start on this trip, remember to approach it with an open mind and a sense of curiosity. Embrace the process, celebrate your growth, and relish in the joy of finding. And above all, respect the deep role that ejaculatory control plays in shaping not just your sexual pleasure, but the very essence of your relationships and your life.

Throughout this guide, we'll uncover the secrets of ejaculation, studying the intricate dance between mind, body, and arousal. We'll discover mindfulness techniques to heighten awareness, sensate focus exercises to increase pleasure, and pelvic floor workouts to improve control. We'll dig into the power of conversation, intimacy, and lifestyle changes, all aimed at empowering you to take charge of your sexual satisfaction.

But let's be clear: this isn't about perfection or show. It's about accepting the trip, celebrating progress, and relishing in the pleasure of finding. Whether you're starting on this trip solo or with a partner by your side, know that you're not alone.

So, dear reader, are you ready to learn the secrets of ejaculation mastery? Are you prepared to start on a path of self-discovery, pleasure, and closeness like never before? If so, let's dive in and explore ten easy-to-follow methods for delaying climax and staying longer in bed. Your road to sexual freedom starts now.

So, whether you're starting on this journey for yourself or with a partner, remember this: ejaculatory control is not just a skill to be learned; it's a gateway to a world of deep closeness, pleasure, and fulfillment. Embrace it, treasure it, and let it lead you on a trip of sexual exploration and self-discovery unlike any other.

**Chapter One:**

**Understanding Ejaculation**

Welcome to the interesting world of ejaculation – a symphony of physiological and psychological factors combining to create one of the most exhilarating experiences known to humans. In this chapter, we'll dive deep into the mechanics of ejaculation, unraveling its secrets and throwing light on the intricate dance between body and mind.

Ejaculation is more than just a physical release; it's a complex interplay of feelings, emotions, and neurochemical reactions. From the flutter of excitement in the pit of your stomach to the surge of pleasure that courses through your veins, every aspect of ejaculation is a testament to the amazing powers of the human body and mind.

So, grab a seat and prepare to start on a trip of exploration and enlightenment. Together, we'll discover the physiological processes that govern ejaculation, from the firing of neurons to the rhythmic contractions of muscles. We'll peer into the depths of the brain, where desire takes root and arousal ignites, forming the very core of our sexual experience.

But understanding ejaculation is not just about dissecting the physical processes at play; it's also about admitting the profound impact of our mental and emotional states. From the whispers of eagerness that quicken our pulse to the waves of relaxation that wash over us in moments of closeness, our thoughts and feelings hold sway over the time and strength of ejaculation.

So, as we start on this path of discovery, let us approach it with wonder and curiosity, eager to unlock the secrets of ejaculation and gain a better understanding of ourselves and our sexuality. Together, we'll peel back the layers of feeling and emotion, unraveling the secrets of ejaculation one thread at a time.

## 1. The Physiological and Psychological Factors Influencing Ejaculation

Ejaculation is like a dance between your body and mind, where every move is guided by a symphony of physiological and psychological factors. Picture it as a delicate balance between the rhythm of your heartbeat and the music of your thoughts, all coming together to create a harmonious experience of happiness and satisfaction.

Physiologically, it's like your body's own orchestra warming up for a show. Nerves send messages like musical notes, setting off a chain reaction that ends in the grand crescendo of ejaculation. Hormones add their own flair, like background musicians harmonizing to improve the experience. And let's not forget about

the muscles, working in perfect synchrony to give the peak.
But the psychological side is just as important. It's like the conductor of this orchestra, directing the tempo and mood of the show. Your feelings set the tone, whether it's the thrill of expectation or the calm of intimacy. Your thoughts act as the score, creating the story of your experience. And your views about yourself and sex play a starring role, affecting how you perceive and respond to pleasure.

By knowing and addressing these factors, you're basically fine-tuning your performance. You're learning to listen to the cues your body and mind are giving you, adjusting the speed and pressure as needed. With practice and care, you can develop greater control over your ejaculatory reaction, lengthening the pleasure and strengthening the connection with your partner.

So, just like a skilled musician perfects their craft through practice and commitment, you too can improve your ability to control ejaculation. And as you do, you'll find yourself opening new levels of sexual happiness and intimacy, creating a symphony of pleasure that echoes long after the final note has faded away.

A.Physiological Factors:
Ejaculation is a symphony of physiological processes organized by the complex workings of the nervous system, hormones, and muscles. At its core lies the

ejaculatory reflex, a complex chain of events caused by sexual stimulation.

Ejaculation is a masterpiece of physiological synchronization, with each component playing a vital part in the production of pleasure and happiness. By knowing the inner workings of this symphony, we can better enjoy the beauty and complexity of our own bodies and lives.

Imagine your body as a highly tuned orchestra, with each instrument playing its part in the music of ejaculation. Let's take a closer look at the bodily factors that organize this complex performance:

1. Neurological Signaling:

When sexual arousal peaks, the brain sends messages to the spinal cord, starting the ejaculatory reflex arc. This flood of nerve signals goes to the muscles of the pelvic floor and reproductive organs, starting ejaculation.

Think of your brain as the director of this orchestra. When you're aroused, it's like the conductor waving the stick, marking the start of the show. Your brain sends messages through a network of nerves to your spinal cord, setting off a chain reaction known as the ejaculatory reflex arc.

This reflex curve is like the artists playing their instruments in perfect harmony. It includes a number of nerve signals traveling from your spinal cord to the muscles in your pelvic floor and reproductive organs.

These impulses kickstart the process of ejaculation,
telling your body to prepare for the grand finish.
2. Hormonal Regulation:
Hormones play a key part in modulating sexual
performance and ejaculation. Testosterone, the main
male sex hormone, affects desire and the production
of seminal fluid, while neurotransmitters like
dopamine and serotonin manage arousal and
pleasure.

Hormones are like the backstage crew working hard
to ensure everything runs smoothly. Testosterone, the
famous hormone, takes center stage, affecting your
libido and the production of seminal fluid. It's like the
main character in the play, setting the tone for the
entire show.

But there are also supporting characters, like
dopamine and serotonin, playing important parts in
the background. Dopamine adds excitement to the
scene, heightening arousal and pleasure, while
serotonin helps manage mood and feelings, keeping
everything in balance.

3. Muscular Contractions:
Finally, we have the muscle contractions – the peak of
the symphony, where everything comes together in a
burst of feeling. Picture your pelvic floor muscles as
the drummers, pounding out a beat that pushes
semen from the seminal vesicles and prostate gland
into the urethra.

During ejaculation, rhythmic movements of the pelvic floor muscles push semen from the seminal vesicles and prostate gland into the urethra. These contractions create the feeling of climax, growing in strength until they reach a peak of their own – the release of semen from the penis. It's like the big finale of a fireworks show, a moment of pure exhilaration and release.

B. Psychological Factors
Psychology is the quiet master directing the music of ejaculation, shaping the time and intensity of your experience. By knowing and controlling the power of your thoughts, feelings, and mental state, you can unlock new levels of pleasure, intimacy, and control in your sexual journey.

1. Arousal and Desire:
Imagine arousal as the flicker of a flame, sparking a firestorm of feelings and wants within you. When you're excited, it's like your body is saying, "Let the show begin!" Your feelings become heightened, and even the smallest touch can send shivers down your spine.  Arousal is the spark that starts the ejaculatory process, fueling desire and increasing sensitivity to sexual stimulation.

Psychological factors like desire, fantasy, and expectation add fuel to this fire. Think of attraction as the magnet that draws you towards your partner, causing a magnetic pull that strengthens your desire. Fantasies act like the script of a steamy romance book, feeding your imagination and increasing your desire. And anticipation? Well, it's like waiting for the curtain to rise on a thrilling show, building tension and excitement with each passing moment.

2. Emotional State:
Emotions play a major part in ejaculation, with stress, anxiety, and performance pressure acting as possible barriers to ejaculatory control. Conversely, feelings of ease, trust, and closeness can promote prolonged arousal and stall ejaculation.

Emotions are the rollercoaster of feelings that can either push you towards ecstasy or derail your journey to pleasure. Stress, nervousness, and performance pressure are like dark clouds rising over the horizon, threatening to rain on your parade. They can tighten your muscles, cloud your thoughts, and sabotage your ability to control ejaculation.

But on the flip side, feelings of rest, trust, and closeness are like rays of sunshine breaking through the clouds. They create a sense of ease and openness, allowing you to let go of fears and fully engage yourself in the moment. When you feel safe and linked with your partner, it's like a weight has been lifted off your back, making it easier to delay ejaculation and prolong pleasure.

3. Cognitive Factors:
Lastly, let's explore the power of your thoughts and beliefs – the quiet builders shaping your sexual

experience. Imagine your thoughts as the storytellers, creating tales that can either strengthen or block your ability to control ejaculation. Our thoughts and ideas about sex and behavior can shape our experience of ejaculation. Negative self-talk or unrealistic standards may lead to premature ejaculation, while positive mantras and mindfulness methods can promote ejaculatory control.

Negative self-talk, like a broken record playing in your mind, can plant seeds of doubt and unease, feeding fears of inadequacy and failure.

But with a change in viewpoint, you can rewrite the script and reclaim your power. Positive mantras become your friends, boosting your confidence and reinforcing beliefs in your ability to master ejaculation. Mindfulness methods act as your guiding light, helping you stay present in the moment and handle the ebbs and flows of desire with grace and ease.

## 2. Role of Arousal, Stimulation, and Mental State in Ejaculation

Arousal, excitement, and mental state are like the three pillars holding the temple of pleasure. When they're in alignment, the trip to ejaculation becomes a symphony of feeling and satisfaction. But when one pillar falters, it can throw off the careful balance of the experience, leaving you adrift in a sea of confusion.

A. Arousal:
Arousal is the electric current that jolts your body awake, like the first rays of dawn creeping over the horizon, slowly nudging you from sleep to waking. It's a slow waking, starting as a mere whisper and crescendoing into a thunderous roar of desire.

Picture yourself as a dormant volcano, hidden in the depths of your being, waiting for the right moment to rise. With each passing moment of arousal, it's like the volcano stirs, sending waves of energy coursing through your blood, sparking a fire within.

As arousal builds, your body becomes a canvas for feeling, drawn with lines of pleasure and desire. Every touch, every kiss, every caress is like a brushstroke, adding to the masterpiece of feeling that spreads before you. Your skin becomes a playground of feeling, living with the tingle of expectation and the warmth of desire.

But excitement is not just a physical feeling; it's also a state of mind. It's the rush of excitement that fills your system when you're faced with an exciting challenge, the surge of happiness that follows times of intense connection with your partner. When you're truly excited, you're fully present in the moment, attuned to every feeling and hungry for more.

Imagine arousal as the spark that starts the fire of passion within you, setting your soul burning with desire. It's the whisper of anticipation that dances across your skin, the spark of joy in the pit of your stomach. Your heart beats faster, your breath quickens, and every cell in your body hums with anticipation as arousal takes hold.

Arousal is the entrance to pleasure, the key that opens the door to a world of feeling and desire. It's a trip of discovery, a dance of passion and hunger that captivates the body and soul alike. And as you welcome the fire of arousal, you open yourself to a world of possibility, where pleasure knows no limits and ecstasy awaits at every turn.

B. Stimulation:
Stimulation is like the gentle breeze that fans the fires of arousal, intensifying the heat and pushing you towards the peak of pleasure. It's the soft caress of a lover's touch, the electric brush of lips against skin, and the rhythmic dance of bodies moving in perfect harmony.

Think of stimulation as the conductor of an orchestra, leading the flow of feeling with expert accuracy. With each touch, each kiss, each stroke, the excitement builds, like a chorus of pleasure reaching towards the heavens. It's a symphony of feeling, with every note and movement adding to the patchwork of pleasure that envelops you.

But stimulation isn't confined to the physical world; it's also a product of the boundless power of thought. Fantasies act as the fuel that feeds the fire, sparking

emotions and fueling desire with each vivid scenario
played out in the mind's eye. Whether it's imagining
yourself in a steamy meeting or fantasizing about
your partner's touch, the mind becomes a playground
of possibility, amplifying the feelings of pleasure and
heightened arousal to new heights.

Stimulation is the bridge between dream and reality,
the conduit through which desire runs from the
depths of the mind to the peaks of physical feeling.
It's a dance of give and take, with each person adding
to the pace and intensity of pleasure. And as
stimulation builds, so too does the expectation of
release, until finally, in a crescendo of ecstasy,
pleasure washes over you like a tidal wave, leaving
you breathless and satisfied.

C. Mental State:
Your mental state is the quiet orchestrator, directing
the music of your sexual experience with a deft hand.
Like the captain of a ship traveling through stormy
seas, your mental state leads you through the
turbulent waters of desire, changing the course of
your arousal and eventually affecting the time and
strength of ejaculation.

Imagine your mental state as the weather patterns
that sweep across the scenery of your mind. When
the skies are clear and the seas are calm, you sail
forth with confidence and ease. You feel relaxed,
grounded, and fully attuned to the present moment,

allowing you to savor each feeling and prolong the pleasure of closeness with your partner.

But just as quickly as a storm can roll in off the horizon, so too can negative feelings like fear, worry, or self-doubt cloud your mental state. These storm clouds throw a shadow over your wants, disrupting the flow of arousal and making it difficult to maintain control over ejaculation. It's like trying to navigate through choppy seas with a foggy mind, unsure of which way to move.

Your mental state is also affected by your views and expectations about sex and performance. Positive beliefs can boost your confidence and empower you to accept pleasure with abandon, while negative beliefs can sow seeds of doubt and inhibit your ability to fully engage in the experience.

Your mental state serves as the lens through which you view and understand your sexual experiences. When it's in sync with your wants, you're able to ride the waves of arousal with grace and skill, prolonging the pleasure and strengthening the connection with your partner. But when storm clouds gather, it's important to recognize them and handle them with compassion and understanding, knowing that clear skies and smooth sailing lie on the other side.

By knowing and respecting the relationship between arousal, stimulation, and mental state, you can develop greater control over your ejaculatory reaction, leading to improved pleasure, closeness, and happiness in your sexual experiences.

## Chapter Two:

## Mindfulness Techniques

Welcome to the world of mindfulness methods – a trip
of self-discovery and strength in the realm of sexual
intimacy. In this chapter, we'll dive into the changing
power of mindfulness practices, giving tools and
strategies to improve self-awareness and control
arousal levels during sexual activity.

Mindfulness is more than just a term; it's a way of
being present in the moment, fully engaged with your
thoughts, feelings, and experiences. Just as a
masterful painter carefully listens to each brushstroke
on the painting, mindfulness asks us to pay attention
to the intricacies of our experience, both in and out of
the bedroom.

As we start on this study, we'll learn how mindfulness
meditation and breathing exercises can serve as
anchors, keeping us in the present moment and
allowing us to manage the ebbs and flows of
excitement with grace and ease. These methods offer
a pathway to greater self-awareness and control,
enabling us to savor the pleasure of intimacy and
strengthen our relationship with ourselves and our
partners.

So, whether you're new to mindfulness or a seasoned
practitioner, join us on this journey as we unlock the

secrets of mindfulness techniques for improved sexual happiness and intimacy. Get ready to develop a deeper knowledge of yourself and your desires, and to start on a road towards greater fulfillment in your sexual experiences.

## 1. Introduction to Mindfulness Practices for Increasing Self-Awareness During Sexual Activity

Welcome to the art of mindfulness in the bedroom – a trip where presence and awareness combine to elevate your sexual adventures to new heights. In this study, we'll discover how mindfulness practices can serve as your trusted allies, leading you towards greater self-awareness and richer intimacy.

Imagine your mind as a vast ocean, with thoughts and feelings ebbing and going like waves. Now, picture mindfulness as the lighthouse standing tall amidst the tumultuous seas, sending its steady beam of awareness to illuminate the depths below. It's about being fully present in the moment, attuned to the sensations, thoughts, and feelings that arise during sexual action.

Mindfulness asks you to become a watcher of your own experience, to watch without judgment as arousal unfolds within you. It's like stepping back from the heat of passion to watch the flames from a distance, allowing you to gain insight into the patterns and rhythms of your desire.

One of the bases of mindfulness practice is meditation, a gentle exercise in focused attention and breath awareness. Just as a sculptor shapes clay with steady hands, meditation allows you to craft your mind, developing a sense of calm and presence that permeates every part of your being. By adding mindfulness meditation into your sexual routine, you can learn to quiet the chatter of the mind, letting go of distractions and submerging yourself fully in the pleasure of the moment.

But awareness is not just about meditation; it's also about harnessing the power of your breath to regulate arousal levels. Imagine your breath as a gentle breeze, leading you through the peaks and dips of feeling with ease and grace. By practicing deep, diaphragmatic breathing during sexual activity, you can learn to manage your arousal, slowing down or ramping up as needed to keep control and increase joy.

Mindfulness techniques offer a pathway to greater self-awareness and strength in the bedroom. By developing present and attention, you can strengthen your relationship with yourself and your partner, savoring each moment of closeness with heightened awareness and appreciation. So, whether you're starting on this journey solo or with a partner by your side, know that mindfulness holds the key to unlocking a world of pleasure and fulfillment in your sexual adventures.

In addition to mindfulness meditation and breath awareness, mindfulness practices cover a wide array of techniques that can be seamlessly blended into your sexual repertoire. Here are a few more:

1. Body Scan: A body scan involves carefully bringing awareness to each part of your body, from head to toe, noticing any feelings, tensions, or areas of pleasure. By performing a body scan during sexual activity, you can become more attuned to the subtle nuances of feeling, improving your ability to handle arousal and joy.

2. Sensory Focus: Mindfulness pushes you to activate all your senses fully. During sexual action, this means giving attention to the feelings of touch, taste, smell, sight, and sound. By immersing yourself in the physical experience of intimacy, you can strengthen your relationship with your partner and amplify feelings of pleasure and happiness.

3. Non-Judgmental Awareness: Mindfulness asks you to watch your events without judgment or connection. Applying this concept to your sexual meetings allows you to let go of standards and performance anxiety, providing a safe and non-threatening space for exploration and vulnerability.

4. Mindful Conversation: Effective conversation is important for developing closeness and understanding with your partner. Mindfulness supports open, honest, and non-defensive conversation, allowing you to voice

your goals, boundaries, and concerns with clarity and compassion.

5. Gratitude Practice: Cultivating an attitude of thanks can improve your respect for the beauty and pleasure of sexual intimacy. Taking a moment to show thanks for your partner, your body, and the experience of connection can strengthen your sense of connection and satisfaction.

6. Progressive Muscle Relaxation: This method includes carefully tensing and then relaxing different muscle groups in the body. By practicing progressive muscle relaxation during sexual action, you can release physical stress and increase awareness of subtle feelings, leading to heightened pleasure and relief.

7. Visualization: This involves thinking of picturing scenes or pictures that evoke feelings of pleasure, connection, and intimacy. By adding visualization methods into your sexual experiences, you can increase arousal, improve feelings, and create a more vivid and immersive experience.

8. Focus on the Present Moment: Mindfulness teaches us to center our attention in the current moment, rather than dwelling on the past or worrying about the future. During sexual activity, focus on the feelings, emotions, and exchanges happening in the here and now, allowing yourself to fully immerse in the experience without distraction.

9. Exploration of Erotic Touch: Take a thoughtful approach to touch by exploring different textures, stresses, and rhythms during sexual action. Pay attention to how each touch feels on your skin and how your body responds, allowing yourself to enjoy the pleasure of intimate relationships with your partner.

10. Single Sensual Exploration: Mindfulness can also be performed during a single sexual action. Take time to study your own body with interest and kindness, noticing sensations without judgment. By cultivating self-awareness and acceptance, you can strengthen your relationship with yourself and enhance solo pleasure encounters.

11. Goal Setting: Before participating in sexual action, take a moment to set a goal for the experience. This could be to focus on pleasure, strengthen connection with your partner, or discover new feelings. By actively setting a purpose, you direct your attention and energy towards a particular result, enhancing mindfulness and presence.

12. Body Awareness Exercises: Practice gentle moves or stretches to connect with your body and improve body awareness. This could include yoga stretches, tai chi moves, or simply stretching and feeling the sensations in your muscles. By tuning into your body's feelings, you can heighten your awareness and presence during sexual action.

13. Erotic Mindfulness: Explore the idea of erotic mindfulness, which includes taking mindfulness techniques directly into your sexual interactions. This could include keeping eye contact with your partner, focusing on the rhythm of your breath, or simply tuning into the feelings of pleasure as they arise. By bringing thoughtful awareness to each moment of closeness, you can strengthen connection and enhance pleasure.

14. Sensate Focus: Sensate focus is a method widely used in sex therapy to improve awareness of physical feelings and boost pleasure. It includes taking turns with your partner to touch and explore each other's bodies, focusing on the feelings without the goal of orgasm. By learning sensate focus, you can improve your understanding of your partner's body and increase shared pleasure.

15. Graded Exposure: If you deal with performance anxiety or fear of closeness, graded exposure can be a helpful mindfulness method. Start by gradually exposing yourself to sexual stimuli or intimate situations in a controlled and helpful setting. With each experience, notice your thoughts and feelings without judgment, allowing yourself to gradually become more comfortable and confident in sexual settings.

By incorporating these mindfulness techniques into your sexual routine, you can develop a greater sense of presence, connection, and satisfaction in your intimate interactions. Whether you're looking to enhance pleasure, improve communication, or increase closeness with your partner, mindfulness offers a powerful toolkit for changing your sexual experiences from ordinary to special.

## 2. Mindfulness Meditation and Breathing Exercises, Powerful Tools for Controlling Arousal Levels During Sexual Activity

A. Mindfulness Meditation:
Imagine yourself sitting in a peaceful garden, surrounded by the gentle rustle of leaves and the sweet smell of flowers. This is the core of mindfulness meditation – a practice of quieting the mind and tuning into the present moment.

To begin awareness meditation, find a comfy position, either sitting or lying down. Close your eyes and bring your attention to your breath, noticing the feeling of each inhale and exhale. As thoughts arise, gently recognize them and let them pass, returning your attention to the breath.

As you continue to focus, you may notice feelings in your body, thoughts in your mind, or emotions arising. Allow these events to simply be, without criticism or attachment. With each breath, develop a sense of calm and presence, allowing yourself to fully engage in the present moment.

Mindfulness meditation can be practiced for as little as a few minutes or as long as you like. The key is consistency – making it a regular part of your habit to reap the rewards of greater self-awareness and mental regulation.

Here's a simple step-by-step guide to mindfulness meditation:

1. Find an Easy Position: Start by finding a quiet and easy place to sit or lie down. You can sit on a chair with your feet flat on the floor or cross-legged on a cushion. If you prefer, you can lie down on your back with your arms by your sides.

2. Close Your Eyes or Lighten Your Gaze: Close your eyes slowly or lighten your gaze by looking downward without focusing on anything in particular. This helps reduce visible distractions and allows you to turn your attention inward.

3. Bring Attention to Your Breath: Begin by bringing your focus to your breath. Notice the sense of the breath as it enters and leaves your body. You can focus on the rise and fall of your chest, the growth and contraction of your belly, or the feeling of air going through your lungs.

4. Be Present with Your Breath: As you continue to breathe, simply watch each inhale and exhale without trying to change or control your breath. Notice the

rhythm and pattern of your breathing, allowing it to move freely and smoothly.

5. Accept Thoughts and Emotions: As thoughts, feelings, and sensations arise in your mind, accept them without judgment or connection. Simply watch them as they come and go, like clouds going through the sky. Then, gently shift your attention back to your breath.

6. Cultivate Acceptance and Compassion: Practice self-compassion and acceptance towards whatever comes during your meditation. If you find your mind drifting or becoming distracted, slowly guide your attention back to your breath with kindness and patience.

7. Continue for a Few Minutes: Set a timer for a few minutes to start with, gradually raising the length as you become more comfortable with the practice. Even just a few minutes of awareness meditation can have a good effect on your mental and emotional well-being.

8. End with Gratitude: When you're ready to end your meditation, take a moment to show gratitude for the time you've committed to yourself. Notice any shifts in your mood, energy, or awareness that may have happened during the exercise.
Mindfulness meditation is a practice – there's no right or wrong way to do it. The most important thing is to approach it with an open mind and a sense of

curiosity and discovery. With constant practice, you'll gradually develop greater self-awareness, mental resilience, and a stronger sense of connection with yourself and the world around you.

B. Breathing Exercises:
Now, let's study the power of breath to control arousal levels during sexual action. Imagine your breath as a gentle wave, rising and falling in rhythm with the ebb and flow of excitement.

One successful breathing practice is called "box breathing." Start by breathing deeply through your nose for a count of four, imagining drawing air into your belly like filling a bag. Hold your breath for a count of four, feeling the fullness and growth in your chest. Then, exhale slowly through your mouth for a count of four, relaxing tightness and letting go of any stress or worry. Finally, hold your breath out for a count of four, feeling a moment of stillness and calm.

Another helpful method is called "progressive relaxation breathing." Begin by breathing deeply and tensing your muscles throughout your body, starting from your toes and making your way up to your head. Hold the tightness for a few seconds, then exhale slowly and release the tension from each muscle group, allowing them to relax fully. With each breath, feel yourself becoming more deeply relaxed and present in your body.

Let's dive deeper into the world of breathing techniques, powerful tools for controlling arousal levels during sexual activity:

1. Box Breathing:
Imagine your breath as a gentle wave, rising and falling in perfect rhythm with the ebb and flow of excitement. Box breathing is like riding this wave, leading you towards a state of calm and centeredness amidst the energy of sexual intimacy.

To learn box breathing, start by finding a comfy position and taking a few deep breaths to settle into your body. Then, follow these steps:

1. Inhale (4 counts): Inhale deeply through your nose for a count of four, thinking that you're filling a balloon in your belly. Feel the air expanding your belly and chest, bringing a sense of fullness and energy into your body.

2. Hold (4 counts): Hold your breath for another count of four, allowing the fullness and expansion to stay in your chest. Feel a sense of stillness and presence wash over you as you pause and gather your attention.

3. Exhale (4 counts): Slowly exhale through your mouth for another count of four, releasing any tightness or worry with each breath out. Imagine letting go of any fears or distractions, allowing yourself to sink deeper into rest.

4. Hold (4 counts): Hold your breath out for a final count of four, feeling a moment of calm and quiet. Notice the space between breaths, allowing yourself to rest in this relaxed state before starting the cycle again.

Continue this pattern of box breathing for several rounds, allowing yourself to become fully engaged in the regular flow of breath. With each cycle, you'll gradually feel a sense of calm and centeredness wash over you, helping to control arousal levels and improve your overall experience of sexual closeness.

2. Progressive Relaxation Breathing:
Progressive relaxation breathing is like a gentle massage for your muscles, helping to release tightness and promote deep rest throughout your body. It's like a trip from tension to tranquility, leading you towards a state of total present and ease.

To perform gradual relaxation breathing, follow these steps:

1. Inhale and Tense (4 counts): Begin by taking a big breath in and tensing the muscles in your toes and feet as hard as you can for a count of four. Feel the tightness spreading through your muscles, causing a sense of alertness and awareness.
2. Exhale and Release (4 counts): Slowly exhale and release the tightness from your toes and feet as you count to four. Feel the muscles relaxing and softening

with each breath out, allowing any leftover tightness
to melt away.

3. Repeat with Each Muscle Group: Continue this
process of inhaling and tensing each muscle group in
your body, from your legs and thighs to your
midsection, chest, arms, shoulders, and neck. With
each exhale, release the tightness from each muscle
group, allowing yourself to sink deeper into rest.

4. Focus on feelings: As you practice gradual
relaxation breathing, pay attention to the feelings in
your body. Notice the difference between tightness
and relaxation, and allow yourself to fully experience
the feeling of relief with each exhale.

5. Deepen Relaxation: With each round of progressive
relaxation breathing, allow yourself to sink deeper
into relaxation, letting go of any lingering tension or
worry. Feel yourself becoming more present and
grounded in your body, ready to fully engage in the
experience of sexual closeness.

Let's explore some additional breathing exercises to
further improve your ability to control excitement
levels during sexual activity:

1. Alternate Nostril Breathing:
Imagine your breath as a bridge between the left and
right parts of your brain, balancing your energy and
creating a feeling of balance and equilibrium.
Alternate nostril breathing, also known as Nadi

Shodhana in yoga, is like a dance of breath, leading you towards a state of balance and peace.

To practice alternate nostril breathing:

- Sit comfortably with your back tall and shoulders loose.

- Use your right hand to close your right nostril and inhale deeply through your left nose for a count of four.

- At the top of your inhale, use your right ring finger to close your left nose and hold your breath for a count of four.

- Release your right thumb and breathe through your right nose for a count of four.

- Inhale through your right nose for a count of four, then close it with your right hand and hold your breath for a count of four.

- Release your left nose and breathe through it for a count of four.

- Repeat this cycle for several times, focused on the smooth and rhythmic flow of breath.

Alternate nostril breathing helps to balance the nervous system, calm the mind, and control arousal levels, making it an excellent practice to add into your sexual routine.

2. Belly Breathing:
Belly breathing, also known as diaphragmatic breathing, is like getting into the power of your body's natural relaxation reaction. It's like giving yourself a big, comfortable hug from the inside out, supporting feelings of calmness and tranquility.

To learn belly breathing:

- Lie down comfortably on your back with your knees bent and feet flat on the floor, or sit in a comfortable position with your neck straight and shoulders relaxed.

- Place one hand on your chest and the other hand on your belly.

- Take a deep breath in through your nose, causing your belly to rise as you fill your lungs with air. Feel your hand on your belly rise with each breath.

- Exhale slowly through your mouth, letting your belly fall as you release the breath. Feel your hand on your belly lower with each breath.
- Continue to breathe deeply and slowly, focused on the rise and fall of your belly with each breath.

Belly breathing helps to trigger the body's relaxation response, reduce stress and tension, and promote a feeling of calm and relaxation, making it an effective method for controlling arousal levels during sexual activity.

3. Sensory Breathing:
Sensory breathing is like tuning into the symphony of feelings in your body, allowing you to fully engage yourself in the present moment and heighten your sense of happiness.

To learn sense breathing:

- Close your eyes and take a few deep breaths to calm yourself.

- As you breathe, focus on a specific feeling in your body that feels pleasurable or soothing. This could be the warmth of your partner's touch, the feeling of your breath going through your body, or the sound of your own heartbeat.

- As you exhale, picture sending your breath to that feeling, amplifying it and allowing it to spread throughout your body.

- Continue to breathe deeply and slowly, focusing on different feelings with each inhale and exhale. Sensory breathing helps to improve your awareness of pleasure and feeling, allowing you to fully engage yourself in the experience of sexual closeness and manage arousal levels more effectively.

By performing mindfulness meditation and breathing exercises, you can learn to control your arousal levels, improve self-awareness, and enhance the pleasure and intimacy of sexual action. So, take a moment to pause, breathe, and connect with the present moment – your body and mind will thank you for it.

**Chapter Three:**

**Sensate Focus Exercises**

Welcome to the world of sensate focus exercises – a journey of research and finding in the realm of sexual pleasure and intimacy. In this chapter, we'll dig into the changing power of sensate focus methods, giving couples a route to enhance their sexual pleasure and delay ejaculation.

Sensate focus is more than just a series of exercises; it's an attitude, a way of approaching closeness with curiosity, openness, and purpose. It's about slowing down, tuning into your body, and enjoying the feelings of touch and connection with your partner.

In this chapter, we'll lead you through a step-by-step process for performing sensate focus exercises as a couple, providing you with tools and techniques to strengthen your connection, heighten your pleasure, and prolong your sexual encounters.

So, whether you're looking to reignite the spark in your relationship, explore new paths of pleasure, or address concerns around premature ejaculation, sensate focus exercises offer a safe, helpful, and effective way to improve your sexual experiences and strengthen your bond with your partner.

Join us on this trip as we unlock the secrets of sensate focus and start on a road towards greater closeness, connection, and happiness in your relationship. Get ready to awaken your senses, ignite your love, and find the true power of touch.

## 1. Explanation of Sensate Focus Techniques

Sensate focus methods are like a roadmap to finding the secret treasures of sexual pleasure and intimacy, leading couples on a journey of exploration and connection. These methods are meant to improve sexual pleasure and delay ejaculation by moving the focus from achieving orgasm to feeling sensual touch and connection with your partner.

Imagine sensate focus as a dance between two souls, where every touch, every caress, is a step towards deeper closeness and connection. It's about slowing down and paying attention to the feelings of touch, allowing yourself to fully engage in the present moment without the pressure of performance or expectation.

Here's how sensate focus methods work to improve sexual pleasure and delay ejaculation:

1. Slowing Down: Sensate focus urges couples to slow down the pace of sexual activity and focus on the trip rather than the goal. By taking the time to explore each other's bodies with curiosity and purpose, you

can heighten arousal and build anticipation, leading to more intense and rewarding experiences.

2. Increasing Sensory Awareness: Sensate focus exercises involve using all five senses – touch, taste, smell, sight, and hearing – to improve pleasure and closeness. By paying attention to the feelings of touch, you can awaken dormant nerve endings and increase pleasure, leading to more satisfying sexual experiences.

3. Exploring Different Touch Techniques: Sensate focus encourages couples to explore with different touch techniques, from light caresses to hard pressure, to discover what feels pleasurable for both partners. By exploring the full range of sensations, you can unlock new paths of pleasure and strengthen your relationship with your partner.

4. Building Emotional Connection: Sensate attention is not just about physical touch; it's also about building emotional closeness and connection with your partner. By engaging in open conversation, sharing wants and limits, and being fully present with each other, you can strengthen your bond and create a helpful and caring environment for sexual exploration.

5. Delaying Ejaculation: By shifting the focus from reaching orgasm to feeling sensual pleasure, sensate focus methods can help delay ejaculation and prolong sexual experiences. By practicing awareness and staying alert to your body's cues, you can better

control arousal levels and increase the pleasure of intimacy with your partner.

6. Mindful Exploration: Sensate focus encourages partners to approach sexual exploration with mindfulness, meaning being fully present and attentive to the feelings and experiences in the moment. By practicing mindfulness during intimate meetings, you can heighten your sense of pleasure, increase sensitivity to touch, and lengthen the time of sexual activity.

7. Slow Progression: Sensate focus exercises often involve a slow progression from non-genital to genital touch, allowing couples to build arousal gradually and become more sensitive to each other's reactions. By starting with non-threatening, non-sexual touch and eventually moving to more intimate contact, couples can ease into the experience and create a sense of safety and comfort.

8. Breath and Relaxation Techniques: Incorporating breathwork and relaxation techniques into sensate focus exercises can help lower anxiety, stress, and performance pressure, all of which can contribute to premature ejaculation. By practicing deep, diaphragmatic breathing and gradual muscle relaxation, couples can promote a state of calmness and ease, allowing for a more enjoyable and longer sexual experience.

9. Communication and Feedback: Effective communication is important for successful sensate focus tasks. Couples are urged to speak freely about their desires, preferences, and limits, and to provide feedback to each other during the activities. By supporting open and honest conversation, couples can improve trust, intimacy, and mutual happiness.

10. Experimentation and Creativity: Sensate focus encourages partners to explore and try with different techniques, positions, and scenarios to find what brings them the most pleasure and happiness. By accepting creativity and spontaneity, couples can keep the spark alive in their relationship and continuously strengthen their sexual connection over time.

11. Practice and Patience: Like any skill, mastering sensate focus methods takes practice and patience. Couples may not experience instant results, but with constant practice and dedication, they can gradually improve their ability to delay ejaculation and enhance sexual pleasure. By tackling sensate focus exercises with a mindset of wonder, discovery, and non-judgment, partners can build a happy and satisfying sexual relationship.

Sensate focus methods offer couples a holistic approach to improving sexual joy and closeness. By accepting the power of touch, conversation, and mindfulness, you can strengthen your relationship with your partner, explore new aspects of pleasure, and create more fulfilling sexual experiences together.

So, let go of expectations, accept the present moment, and start on a journey of sensual discovery with your partner.

Sensate focus methods are like the secret ingredients in the recipe for a successful and deeply satisfying sexual relationship. They're a set of exercises meant to help couples improve closeness, strengthen connection, and explore pleasure in a whole new way.

Imagine sensate focus as a treasure map taking you and your partner on a journey of discovery through the scenery of your bodies. It's like going on a thrilling journey where every touch, every caress, holds the potential for newfound pleasure and excitement.

Here's a better look at what sensate focus methods entail:

1. Non-Genital Touch Exploration: Sensate focus often starts with non-genital touch exploration, where partners take turns gently touching each other's bodies without focusing on arousal or reaching pleasure. This can include discovering different textures, temperatures, and feelings, like feather-light touches, soothing strokes, or even fun tickles.

2. Mindful Touch: Sensate focus encourages partners to approach touch with mindfulness, meaning being fully present and attentive to the feelings and experiences in the moment. It's about slowing down

and savoring each touch, noticing the nuances of pleasure and connection that appear with each encounter.

3. Progressive Sensual Escalation: As partners become more comfortable with non-genital touch, sensate focus routines may progress to include more close and sensual contact. This could involve discovering erogenous zones, like the neck, chest, and inner thighs, and playing with different levels of pressure, speed, and intensity.

4. Genital Exploration: Eventually, sensate attention may lead to genital exploration, where partners gently touch and explore each other's genital areas with curiosity and care. The focus here is on feeling and connection rather than performance or reaching orgasm, allowing partners to strengthen their closeness and knowledge of each other's bodies.

5. Communication and Feedback: Throughout the sensate focus process, communication is key. Partners are urged to freely share their desires, preferences, and limits, and to provide feedback to each other about what feels pleasurable and what doesn't. This open dialogue promotes trust, intimacy, and mutual happiness.

6. Relaxation and Breathwork: Sensate focus often incorporates relaxation methods, such as deep breathing and gradual muscle relaxation, to help partners release stress, reduce anxiety, and improve

pleasure. By learning relaxation methods together,
partners can create a calm and loving environment for
discovery and intimacy.

7. Emotional link: Beyond physical touch, sensate
focus also aims to strengthen emotional link between
partners. By engaging in personal and vulnerable
moments of touch and discovery, couples can
strengthen their bond, improve intimacy, and create a
greater sense of closeness and trust.

In essence, sensate focus methods are about
welcoming curiosity, fun, and open-mindedness as
you and your partner start on a journey of sexual
exploration and discovery. It's about tuning into each
other's bodies, hearts, and minds, and creating a
place where pleasure, connection, and closeness can
thrive. So, let your senses be your guide, and let the
magic of sensate focus turn your relationship into a
haven of love, desire, and satisfaction.

## 2. Step-by-step Guide to Sensate Focus Exercises for Couples

Let's start on a step-by-step journey through sensate
focus exercises for couples, where pleasure and
closeness await at every touch:

A. Setting the Scene:
Begin by making a comfortable and inviting place
where you and your partner can fully relax and
connect without distractions. Dim the lights, play soft

music, and perhaps light some candles to set the scene for closeness and exploring.

Setting the scene is like putting down the base for a beautiful picture – it's about creating the perfect backdrop for your personal journey with your partner. Here's how to set the scene for sensate focus exercises:

1. Create a Comfortable Space: Find a cozy and private space where you and your mate can fully relax and feel at ease. This could be your bedroom, sitting room, or any place where you both feel safe and relaxed.

2. Dim the Lights: Soft, gentle lighting can help create a warm and private environment. Dim the ceiling lights and opt for softer, more natural lighting sources like lamps, string lights, or candles. The soft glow will cast a sweet and sexual vibe over the room.

3. Play Soft Music: Choose soothing and melodic music that improves relaxation and sets the scene for closeness. Instrumental music, ambient sounds, or slow-tempo songs are ideal for creating a quiet and tranquil mood. Let the music fill the space and bring you into a state of relaxation and connection.

4. Light Candles: Candles add a bit of beauty and sensuality to the atmosphere. Choose scented candles with smells like lavender, jasmine, or vanilla to create a calming and sensual aroma. Place them carefully

around the room to create a soft, flickering glow that adds warmth and closeness to the space.

5. Remove Distractions: Create a distraction-free atmosphere by turning off electronic devices, such as phones, tablets, and computers. This allows you and your partner to fully focus on each other and the experience at hand without interruptions or distractions.

6. Set the Goal: Before you begin, take a moment to set the goal for your sensate focus exercise. This could be to strengthen your relationship with your partner, explore new paths of pleasure, or simply enjoy each other's company in a relaxed and intimate setting. By setting a clear goal, you and your partner connect your energies and create a shared sense of purpose for the experience.

By setting the scene in this way, you create a nurturing and helpful environment that supports relaxation, intimacy, and connection between you and your partner. So, dim the lights, play some soft music, light the candles, and get ready to start on a trip of sensuality and exploration together.

B. Agree on Intentions:
Before getting into the routines, take a moment to discuss your goals and wishes with your partner. Be open and honest about what you hope to experience and what limits you want to set. This sets the stage

for trust, conversation, and mutual respect throughout the process.

Agreeing on intentions is like setting sail on a trip with a clear destination in mind – it ensures that you and your partner are on the same page and ready to start on the adventure together. Here's how to agree on goals before getting into sensate focus exercises:

1. Open Communication: Start by making a safe and non-judgmental place where you and your partner can openly share your thoughts, feelings, and desires. Encourage each other to speak honestly and truly, without fear of judgment or criticism.

2. Share Your Hopes and Desires: Take turns sharing what you hope to experience during the sensate focus activities. This could include desires for greater intimacy, discovery of new feelings, or simply a desire to connect with your partner on a deeper level. Be clear and open about what you're looking for from the experience.

3. Establish Boundaries: Discuss any bounds or limits that you want to set for the activities. This could include limits around certain types of touch, specific parts of the body, or any activities that you're not okay with. Respect each other's limits and agree to respect them throughout the process.

4. Clarify Goals: Be clear about your goals for the tasks and what you hope to achieve as a couple.

Whether it's enhancing intimacy, better communication, or finding new avenues of pleasure, make sure you're both on the same page about what you want to get out of the experience.

5. Listen and Support: Take the time to actively listen to your partner's goals and wishes, and support their feelings and experiences. Show empathy and understanding, even if you don't share the same goals or limits. This helps to build trust and equal respect between you and your partner.

6. Find Common Ground: Look for areas of common ground and similar goals that you can work towards together. Focus on the aspects of the experience that excite and inspire both of you, and use them as a basis for your journey of exploration and connection.

7. Agree on a Plan: Once you've reviewed your goals and desires, come to a joint understanding on how you want to continue with the sensate focus exercises. This could involve making specific goals, establishing a schedule, or describing the activities you want to explore together.

By agreeing on goals before diving into the exercises, you and your partner lay the groundwork for a positive and satisfying experience. You build trust, foster open communication, and create a shared sense of purpose that leads you through the journey of pleasure and discovery together. So, take the time to discuss your intentions, listen to each other's

wishes, and start on the journey with a sense of
clarity and mutual understanding.
C. Non-Genital Touch Exploration:
Non-genital touch exploration is like going on a trip of
discovery, where every caress, stroke, and touch
leads to new sensations and heightened pleasure.
Here's how to start:

1. Create a Comfortable Environment: Ensure that
you and your partner are in a comfortable and
relaxing place where you both feel at ease. Dim the
lights, play soft music, and remove any distractions to
set the stage for closeness and connection.

2. Take Turns Exploring: Begin by taking turns
exploring each other's bodies with non-genital touch.
Start with one partner as the giver and the other as
the receiver, then switch roles. This provides a
balanced and reciprocal relationship where both
partners have the chance to give and receive
pleasure.

3. Gentle Caresses and Stroking: Use your hands,
fingers, and cheeks to gently caress and stroke your
partner's body. Start with broad, wide movements to
warm up the skin, then gradually shift to lighter, more
delicate touches. Pay attention to your partner's
reactions and change your touch accordingly.

4. Relaxing Massages: Incorporate relaxing massages
into your non-genital touch research. Use long,
flowing strokes to knead and move your partner's

muscles, focusing on areas of tightness and stress. Experiment with different massage methods, such as Swedish, deep tissue, or shiatsu, to find what feels best for both of you.

5. Playful Tickles: Add an element of fun and spontaneity to your touch discovery by adding playful tickles. Gently run your fingers along your partner's skin, exploring sensitive areas like the back of the neck, underarms, and sides. Pay attention to your partner's response and laughter, and enjoy the sense of light-heartedness and connection that comes with fun touch.

6. Sensory Tools: Enhance the sensory experience by adding tools like feathers, silk scarves, or soft brushes into your touch study. Use these props to produce different textures and feelings on your partner's skin, further heightening their arousal and pleasure.

7. Speak and Connect: Throughout the non-genital touch exploration, speak freely with your partner and stay attentive to their reactions. Use verbal and non-verbal cues to describe what feels good and what doesn't, and encourage your partner to do the same. This provides a sense of connection and intimacy as you handle the journey of touch together.

By starting with non-genital touch discovery, you and your partner lay the basis for greater intimacy and connection. You awaken each other's senses, spark desire and pleasure, and set the stage for further

discovery and arousal. So, take your time, savor the
feelings, and enjoy the journey of touch discovery
with your partner.

D. Mindful Touch:
Mindful touch is like a dance of awareness, where
every feeling is felt deeply and every moment is
savored fully. Here's how to learn mindful touch with
your partner:

1. Be current: Before you begin, take a moment to
center yourself and bring your mind to the current
moment. Let go of any distractions or problems and
focus solely on your partner and the feelings of touch.

2. Start Slowly: Begin by gently touching your
partner's skin with your fingers, hands, or the back of
your hand. Notice the feel of their skin, the warmth of
their body, and the way their muscles respond to your
touch. Take your time and allow yourself to fully
experience each feeling.

3. Use All Your Senses: Engage all your senses as you
explore your partner's body. Notice the smell of their
skin, the sound of their breath, and the sight of their
responses to your touch. Allow yourself to become
fully engaged in the physical experience of touch.

4. Stay Curious: Approach each touch with a sense of
wonder and discovery. Notice how your partner reacts
to different types of touch and try with changing

pressure, speed, and intensity. Be open to finding new ways of causing pleasure and connection.

5. Talk: Throughout the practice of mindful touch, talk freely with your partner about what feels pleasurable and what doesn't. Use verbal and non-verbal cues to express your wants and tastes, and encourage your partner to do the same. This provides a sense of mutual understanding and improves the connection between you.

6. Stay in the Moment: Resist the desire to let your mind roam or become sidetracked during the practice of focused touch. Instead, focus your attention fully on your partner and the feelings of touch, allowing yourself to be fully present and involved in the experience.

7. Show Thanks: At the end of your mindful touch session, take a moment to show thanks to your partner for sharing this intimate experience with you. Acknowledge the pleasure and connection that you've both experienced and show appreciation for the chance to strengthen your bond through touch.

By learning mindful touch with your partner, you develop a deeper sense of closeness, connection, and presence in your relationship. You learn to savor each moment, value the beauty of touch, and improve your knowledge of each other's wants and preferences. So, accept the practice of focused touch and allow it to improve your relationship in deep and meaningful ways.

E. Progressive Sensual Escalation:
Progressive sexual increase is like a gentle crescendo, where the intensity of pleasure builds slowly and steady, leading to greater closeness and connection. Here's how to discover increasing sensual escalation with your partner:

1. Build on Non-Genital Touch: Start by continuing to explore each other's bodies with non-genital touch, gradually raising the level of sensuality and closeness. Use the techniques you've already tried, such as gentle touches, soothing massages, and fun tickles, to build arousal and anticipation.

2. Focus on Erogenous Zones: As you both become more comfortable with non-genital touch, begin to explore erogenous zones – areas of the body that are particularly sensitive to touch and can trigger pleasant feelings. These may include the neck, chest, inner legs, ears, and nipples. Experiment with different types of touch and pressure to discover what feels most pleasurable for both you and your partner.

3. Vary Pressure, Speed, and Intensity: Explore different levels of pressure, speed, and intensity as you touch and caress each other's erogenous zones. Use light, feather-like touches to tease and titillate, and harder, more deliberate strokes to increase arousal. Pay attention to your partner's reactions and change your touch accordingly to maximize pleasure.

4. Encourage Communication: Throughout the process of gradual sensual escalation, encourage your partner to speak freely about what feels pleasant and what doesn't. Use verbal and non-verbal cues to voice your own wants and preferences, and be receptive to your partner's comments. This open conversation produces a sense of trust, intimacy, and mutual satisfaction as you discover together.

5. Be Receptive to Feedback: Be receptive and responsive to your partner's feedback, adjusting your touch and method based on their tastes and comfort level. Respect their limits and tastes, and create a safe and supportive place for discovery and expression. Remember that happiness is relative, and what feels good for one person may not feel the same for another.

6. Enjoy the Trip: Above all, remember to enjoy the trip of increasing sexual escalation with your partner. Focus on the pleasure and connection you share, and enjoy each moment of intimacy and discovery. Embrace the chance to strengthen your bond and enhance your sexual relationship as you discover new levels of sensuality together.

By exploring gradual sensual escalation with your partner, you can strengthen your closeness, enhance your connection, and discover new paths of pleasure and satisfaction. So, take your time, speak openly, and enjoy the trip of exploration and discovery together.

F. Genital Exploration:
Genital exploration is like going on a sacred trip of intimacy and connection, where every touch is led by love, curiosity, and mutual respect. Here's how to approach sexual play with your partner:

1. Mutual Readiness: Before moving to genital probing, ensure that both you and your partner feel comfortable, relaxed, and ready to take this step together. Check in with each other to measure readiness and share any worries or reservations you may have.

2. Create a Safe Space: Establish a safe and welcoming environment for genital play, free from distractions or delays. Dim the lights, play soft music, and create a sense of closeness and privacy that allows you to fully focus on each other and the experience at hand.

3. Focus on Sensation and Connection: Shift your focus from performance or reaching orgasm to simply enjoying the pleasures and strengthening your connection with your partner. Approach genital play with a sense of wonder, openness, and respect for each other's bodies.

4. Use Your Hands, Fingers, and Lips: Use your hands, fingers, and lips to explore each other's private areas with kindness, care, and respect. Start with light, teasing touches and gradually increase pressure and strength as desire builds. Experiment with different

touches, kisses, and techniques to discover what feels pleasurable for both you and your partner.

5. Talk Freely: Throughout genital discovery, talk freely and honestly with your partner about what feels pleasant and what doesn't. Use verbal and non-verbal cues to voice your desires, preferences, and limits, and encourage your partner to do the same. This open conversation promotes trust, intimacy, and mutual satisfaction.

6. Be Receptive to Your Partner's Cues: Pay close attention to your partner's verbal and non-verbal cues during genital exploration, and be receptive to their wants and comfort level. Respect their limits and tastes, and change your touch and method accordingly to ensure a pleasant and enjoyable experience for both of you.

7. Enjoy the Journey: Above all, remember to enjoy the trip of genital exploring with your partner. Focus on the pleasure and connection you share, and enjoy each moment of intimacy and discovery. Embrace the chance to strengthen your bond and improve your sexual connection as you explore new levels of passion and closeness together.

By approaching genital exploration with interest, openness, and respect, you can strengthen your intimacy, enhance your connection, and discover new paths of pleasure and happiness with your partner.

So, take your time, speak openly, and enjoy the trip
of exploration and discovery together.

G. Relaxation and Breathwork:
Relaxation and breathwork are like the secret
ingredients that add a special flavor to your private
times with your partner. Here's an easier way to
understand and perform them:

1. Deep Breathing: Take slow, deep breaths together,
filling your lungs with air like you're stretching a
bubble. Imagine your breath moving in and out easily,
like the gentle waves of the ocean. As you breathe
deeply, feel the stress melting away from your body,
leaving you feeling cool and relaxed.

2. Sync Your Breaths: Sync your breath with each
touch and movement, like you're dancing to a slow,
steady beat. Inhale together as you lean in for a
caress, and exhale as you release and rest. This helps
you stay linked with each other and improves the
pleasure of your touch.

3. Progressive Muscle Relaxation: Start by tensing and
then releasing each muscle group in your body, one at
a time. Begin with your toes and work your way up to
your head, stiffening each muscle group for a few
seconds before letting go. Feel the stress melting
away with each breath, leaving you feeling light,
loose, and completely at ease.

4. Sink into Relaxation: Allow yourselves to sink deeper into relaxation with each breath and each touch. Let go of any fears or distractions, and fully engage yourselves in the present moment. Feel the warmth of your partner's touch and the soothing beat of your breaths, as you bask in the blissful feeling of relaxation and connection.

By practicing relaxation and breathwork together, you create a peaceful and harmonious environment that improves the pleasure and closeness of your shared moments. So, take a deep breath, rest, and enjoy the journey of bonding and intimacy with your partner.

H. Emotional Connection:
Emotional connection is like building a strong link with your partner, where you feel close, understood, and encouraged. Here's an easier way to strengthen your emotional connection:

1. Share Your Feelings: Take the time to talk freely and honestly with your partner about how you're feeling. Share your thoughts, dreams, and fears, and listen carefully to what they have to say. This develops a sense of understanding and connection between you.

2. Be Vulnerable: Don't be afraid to show your vulnerable side and share your feelings authentically. Let your partner see the real you, flaws and all, and trust that they will love and accept you just as you

are. This strengthens the bond between you and
promotes greater intimacy.

3. Create a Safe Space: Make sure you create a safe
and helpful environment where you both feel
comfortable sharing yourselves without fear of
judging or rejection. Be respectful of each other's
feelings and make a place where you can be open and
honest with each other.

4. Celebrate Each Other: Take the time to celebrate
and respect each other's bodies and the pleasure you
share together. Express thanks for the love, intimacy,
and bond you experience, and show respect for the
little things your partner does to make you happy.

By focusing on emotional connection, you can improve
the bond between you and your partner, enhance your
intimacy, and create a more fulfilling and enjoyable
relationship. So, take the time to connect personally
with your partner and enjoy the deep sense of
connection and understanding that comes with it.

I. Reflection and Integration:
Reflection and merging are like looking back on a trip
you've taken together and working out what you've
learned along the way. Here's an easier way to
understand this:

1. Talk About Your Experience: Take some time to
chat with your partner about what you just did. Share
how you felt during the tasks, what you liked or didn't

like, and any new things you learned about each other.

2. Think About the Future: Discuss how you can keep using these techniques in your sex life. Maybe you want to try them again sometime, or maybe you have other ideas for how to keep things fun and exciting in the bedroom.

3. Remember It's a Journey: Understand that studying your sexuality is a constant process. There's always more to learn and find, so don't rush it. Take your time, keep talking with your partner, and enjoy the ride together.

By thinking about your experiences and integrating what you've learned into your relationship, you can keep getting closer and enjoying each other's company even more. So, keep talking, keep trying, and keep having fun together!

J. Practice and Enjoyment:
Practice and happiness are like learning to play a new game – the more you do it, the better you get, and the more fun you have. Here's an easier way to understand this:

1. Keep Trying: Sensate attention exercises aren't something you just do once and then forget about. They're like a fun game you can keep coming back to with your partner whenever you want to feel closer and more linked.

2. Stay Curious: Approach each time you do the exercises with a sense of wonder and energy, like you're discovering uncharted territory together. Keep trying new things and seeing what you both enjoy the most.

3. Have Fun: Remember that the point of doing these routines is to have fun and feel good together. Don't think too much about getting everything right – just enjoy each other's company and the pleasure you share.

By performing sensate focus exercises regularly and approaching them with a sense of joy and curiosity, you can improve your bond with your partner and keep the spark alive in your relationship for years to come. So, keep working, keep enjoying, and keep loving each other!

Sensate focus exercises offer couples an organized and fun approach to improving pleasure and closeness in their relationship. By following these steps and embracing the spirit of exploration and connection, you can open new dimensions of pleasure, strengthen your bond with your partner, and build a happy and satisfying sexual relationship together. So, let the trip begin, and may each touch be a step towards better love, passion, and bond with your partner.

# Chapter Four:

## Pelvic Floor Exercises: Strengthening Your Core for Sexual Mastery

Welcome to the world of pelvic floor movements, where the key to unlocking ejaculatory control lies within the core of your body. Just like a strong base supports a sturdy house, your pelvic floor muscles provide the essential framework for sexual mastery and enhanced pleasure.

In this trip, we'll dig into the intricate network of muscles nestled deep within your pelvis and discover their crucial role in ejaculatory control. From knowing the anatomy of the pelvic floor to learning the art of kegel exercises and other workouts, we'll equip you with the tools and skills to strengthen your core and take control of your sexual experience.

So, prepare to start on a transformative trip that will not only improve your sexual prowess but also deepen your relationship with your body and your partner. Get ready to release the power of your pelvic floor and elevate your sexual happiness to new heights.

## 1. The Pelvic Floor Muscles and Their Role in Ejaculatory Control

The pelvic floor muscles are like the unsung heroes of your body, quietly working behind the scenes to support important processes and ensure everything stays in its proper place. Located at the base of your pelvis, these muscles form a hammock-like structure that supports your bladder, rectum, and, yes, even your sexual organs.

Now, let's look a little deeper into their role in ejaculatory control. Picture a set of muscles that wrap around the base of your penis like a snug little hug. These muscles play a crucial role in regulating the flow of urine, controlling bowel movements, and, you got it, managing ejaculation.

During sexual arousal, these muscles tighten and relax in a coordinated dance, helping to keep an erection and control the time of ejaculation. When you're on the brink of climax, these muscles kick into high gear, squeezing tightly to delay the release of semen and lengthen the pleasure of the moment.

But here's where things get really interesting: just like any other muscle in your body, your pelvic floor muscles can be strengthened and trained through specific workouts. By participating in regular pelvic floor workouts, like kegel movements, you can improve the strength and endurance of these muscles, leading to better ejaculatory control and more satisfying sexual experiences.

So, think of your pelvic floor muscles as your secret tool in the quest for sexual control. With a little commitment and some smart training, you can unlock their full potential and take your bedroom performance to new heights.

Let's dive even deeper into the complex world of pelvic floor muscles and their role in ejaculatory control:

1. Anatomy of the Pelvic Floor: Imagine your pelvic floor muscles as a strong network of tissues and fibers that span the bottom of your pelvis, like a sturdy bed. These muscles include the pubococcygeus (PC) muscle, the bulbocavernosus muscle, and the ischiocavernosus muscle, among others. Together, they form a strong foundation that supports your pelvic organs and helps manage different bodily processes.

2. Ejaculatory Control: When it comes to sexual function, the pelvic floor muscles play a key part in ejaculatory control. As arousal builds during sexual action, these muscles tighten rhythmically, helping to keep an erection and prevent ejaculation. By contracting these muscles at the right time, you can successfully "hold back" ejaculation and lengthen the pleasure of the experience.

3. Strength and Stamina: Like any muscle in your body, the pelvic floor muscles can benefit from regular exercise to improve their strength and stamina. Kegel movements, which involve tightening and relaxing the pelvic floor muscles, are a popular and effective way to strengthen these muscles. By adding kegel exercises into your routine, you can improve your ejaculatory control and enhance sexual happiness.

4. Benefits Beyond the Bedroom: Strengthening your pelvic floor muscles isn't just about better sex – it also offers a range of other health benefits. A strong pelvic floor can help avoid urinary incontinence, support pelvic organ health, and even improve balance and stability. So, by investing in pelvic floor exercises, you're not just improving your sexual performance – you're investing in your general well-being.

5. Coordination and Time: Ejaculatory control isn't just about the strength of your pelvic floor muscles; it's also about their coordination and time. During sexual excitement, these muscles work in harmony with other muscle groups, nerves, and hormonal messages to control the time of ejaculation. By improving your ability to coordinate the contractions of your pelvic floor muscles, you can take greater control over your ejaculatory reaction.

6. Mind-Body Connection: The link between the pelvic floor muscles and ejaculatory control goes beyond mere physical strength and coordination – it also includes a strong mind-body connection. By

developing attention and awareness of your pelvic floor muscles, you can learn to tune into subtle sensations and cues that signal approaching ejaculation. This heightened awareness allows you to intervene and change your pelvic floor muscle action to delay ejaculation as desired.

7. Individual Variability: It's important to understand that the experience of ejaculatory control changes from person to person. Factors such as age, general health, and individual physiology can affect the strength and function of the pelvic floor muscles, as well as the ability to control ejaculation. Additionally, national views, upbringing, and personal ideas about sex and sexuality may also play a role in shaping an individual's experience of ejaculatory control.

8. Holistic Approach: Achieving good ejaculatory control includes more than just strengthening the pelvic floor muscles – it takes a holistic approach that handles physical, psychological, and social factors. In addition to pelvic floor movements, methods such as awareness, calmness, talking with your partner, and trying different sexual techniques can all contribute to better ejaculatory control and increased sexual pleasure.

9. Lifestyle Factors: Beyond exercise and physical health, lifestyle factors can also impact the function of pelvic floor muscles and ejaculatory control. Factors such as food, hydration, stress levels, and sleep quality can all impact pelvic floor health and sexual

performance. By choosing a healthy lifestyle that includes regular exercise, balanced nutrition, adequate hydration, stress management techniques, and sufficient rest, people can support the optimal function of their pelvic floor muscles and improve ejaculatory control.

10. Medical Conditions: Certain medical conditions, such as prostate problems, pelvic floor issues, and neurological diseases, can affect pelvic floor muscle function and ejaculatory control. Seeking proper medical care and treating underlying health problems is important for optimizing pelvic floor health and sexual function. Medical treatments, physical therapy, and lifestyle changes may be suggested to address pelvic floor dysfunction and improve ejaculatory control.

11. Age-Related Changes: As people age, changes in hormone levels, muscle tone, and overall health can affect pelvic floor function and ejaculatory control. While aging is a normal process, adopting healthy living habits and adding pelvic floor movements into one's routine can help reduce age-related changes and maintain optimal sexual function and happiness.

12. Sexual Conversation: Open and honest conversation with sexual partners is important for optimizing ejaculatory control and enhancing sexual satisfaction. By sharing preferences, wants, and concerns with their partners, people can work together to explore techniques and strategies that

promote mutual happiness and satisfaction. Additionally, creating a helpful and understanding environment can help ease performance anxiety and promote relaxation, which are conducive to better ejaculatory control.

The pelvic floor muscles are like the heart of sexual function, supporting everything from erection strength to ejaculatory control. Understanding the multifaceted nature of pelvic floor muscles and their role in ejaculatory control requires consideration of various factors, including lifestyle, medical conditions, age-related changes, sexual communication, their anatomy and role in sexual function, and by incorporating targeted exercises into your routine, you can unlock their full potential and enjoy a more satisfying and fulfilling sex life.

## 2. Demonstration of Kegel Exercises and Other Pelvic Floor Workouts to Strengthen Control

1. Kegel Exercises:
Kegel movements are like training for your pelvic floor muscles – they help strengthen and tone these muscles, leading to better control over ejaculation. Here's how to do them:

A. Find Your Pelvic Floor Muscles:
Finding your pelvic floor muscles is like finding hidden treasure – once you spot them, you'll have the key to unlocking better control and happiness in your sex life. Here's an easier way to find them:

1. Stop the Flow: When you're peeing, try to stop the flow of urine halfway through. The muscles you use to do this are your pelvic floor muscles.

2. Hold in Gas: Another way to find your pelvic floor muscles is to pretend you're trying to hold in gas. The muscles you tighten to do this are also your pelvic floor muscles.

By practicing these simple tricks, you'll become more familiar with your pelvic floor muscles and be ready to start on the trip to stronger control and greater pleasure in the bedroom.

B. Contracting and keeping your pelvic floor muscles is like giving them a little squeeze, just like you would if you were trying to hold in pee. Here's a better way to do it:

1. Squeeze Tight: Once you've found your pelvic floor muscles, tighten them up by squeezing, as if you're trying to stop yourself from peeing. It's like giving them a gentle hug.

2. Hold It: Keep the squeeze going for a few seconds, like you're holding your breath underwater. Try to hold it straight and strong.

3. Let Go: After a few seconds, remove the squeeze and let your muscles relax fully. It's like letting out a deep breath after holding it in for a while.

By performing this squeeze-and-hold method regularly, you'll strengthen your pelvic floor muscles and improve your control over ejaculation, leading to more satisfying sexual experiences.

C. Repeat: Try doing the squeezing and holding practice about 10 to 15 times in a row. Each time you squeeze, hold it tight for about 3 to 5 seconds, like you're counting to yourself slowly. As your muscles get stronger, you can try holding for longer each time, just like pulling bigger weights at the gym when you get stronger.

2. Reverse Kegels:
Reverse kegels are like the opposite of regular kegel exercises – instead of squeezing, you're focused on resting and letting go. Here's a better way to do it:

Relax and Lengthen: Take a big breath in, then breathe out slowly and fully. As you breathe out, imagine pushing down and out with your pelvic floor muscles, like you're trying to rest and stretch them out. It's like letting out a big sigh and feeling all the stress melt away.

Hold and Release: After you've pushed down gently with your pelvic floor muscles, hold that relaxed feeling for a few seconds. Then, slowly let go and come back to a normal, relaxed position. Focus on the feeling of letting all the tightness go and allowing your pelvic floor muscles to fully relax. It's like taking a big breath and feeling your body open up.

3. Bridge Pose:
Bridge pose is a yoga-inspired workout that targets the pelvic floor muscles and helps improve strength and flexibility. Here's how to do it:

1. Lie on Your Back: Start by lying down on your back with your legs bent and your feet flat on the floor. Make sure your feet are about hip-width apart and your arms are sitting easily by your sides.

2. Lift Your Hips: Take a deep breath in, then as you exhale, press strongly into your feet and lift your hips up towards the sky. Imagine pushing the floor away with your feet as you lift your hips. Keep your shoulders and neck relaxed on the ground.

3. Engage Your Pelvic Floor: While you're in the lifted position, focus on working your pelvic floor muscles. Imagine drawing your pelvic floor muscles upward towards your belly button. It's like you're pulling them up and in towards your body.

4. Hold and Lower: Hold the lifted pose for a few breaths, feeling the strength and activation in your pelvic floor muscles. Then, slowly lower your hips back down to the ground as you breathe. Take a moment to rest and relax before continuing the movement.

5. Repeat: Aim to do several rounds of the Bridge Pose, focusing on keeping proper form and working your pelvic floor muscles throughout the action. As you get more comfortable with the exercise, you can gradually increase the number of repetitions and the length of each hold.

By practicing the Bridge Pose daily, you'll not only strengthen your pelvic floor muscles but also improve your general strength, flexibility, and stability. Plus, it's a great way to connect with your body and ease stress in your lower back and hips.

4. Squats:
Squats are a compound workout that involves multiple muscle groups, including the pelvic floor muscles. Here's how to do them:

1. Stand Tall: Begin by standing up straight with your feet about hip-width apart. Your toes can be slightly turned outwards for balance.

2. Lower Your Body: Take a deep breath in, then slowly bend your knees and lower your body down as if you're sitting back into a chair. Keep your shoulders high and your back straight as you lower down. It's important to keep your weight in your feet and your knees lined with your toes to avoid strain.

3. Engage Your Pelvic Floor: While you're in the squat pose, think that you're pulling your pelvic floor muscles upward towards your belly button. This

connection helps to support your lower body and keep stability. Hold this contraction as you breathe and prepare to stand back up.

4. Return to Upright: Exhale as you push through your heels and lift your legs to return to the upright position. Press your hips forward slightly as you stand up tall again. Remember to keep your core engaged and maintain good balance throughout the movement.

5. Repeat: Aim to do several repeats of squats, focusing on keeping proper form and working your pelvic floor muscles with each repetition. Start with a few repetitions and gradually raise the number as you become more comfortable with the exercise.

By adding squats into your normal workout routine, you'll not only strengthen your lower body muscles but also engage your pelvic floor muscles for better stability and support. Plus, squats are a useful exercise that can help improve your general strength and movement for daily tasks.

Here are some extra exercises that can help strengthen your pelvic floor muscles, improve control over ejaculation, and boost sexual satisfaction:

1. Dead Bug Exercise:
By performing the Dead Bug Exercise daily, you can strengthen your core muscles, including the pelvic floor, and improve stability in your spine, which can

contribute to better control over ejaculation and improved sexual satisfaction.

1. Starting Position: Lie on your back on a soft surface, like a yoga mat or couch. Bend your knees so that your feet are flat on the floor, hip-width apart. Extend your arms straight up towards the sky, hands facing each other.

2. Engage Your Core: Take a deep breath in and slowly draw your belly button towards your back to engage your core muscles. This helps stabilize your back throughout the activity.

3. Lower One Arm and Leg: As you breathe, slowly lower your right arm towards the floor behind your head, while equally lowering your left leg towards the ground. Keep your lower back pressed into the floor to keep a stable spine position.

4. Return to Starting Position: Inhale as you bring your right arm and left leg back to the starting position, with your arm extended towards the sky and your knee bent at a 90-degree angle. Keep your center engaged throughout the movement.

5. Repeat on the Other Side: Exhale as you lower your left arm and right leg towards the ground, then inhale as you return to the starting position. Alternate sides for the appropriate number of repeats.

6. Focus on Form: Pay attention to keeping a steady and controlled movement throughout the practice. Avoid raising your lower back or moving your head and shoulders off the ground. Keep your core muscles engaged to support your spine and protect your lower back.

2. Plank Variations:
Planks are excellent for working the entire core, including the pelvic floor muscles. Try versions such as forearm planks, side planks, and planks with leg lifts to test your core stability and improve your pelvic floor muscles.

A. Forearm Plank:
- Start by lying face down on the floor with your arms bent and directly under your shoulders.
- Lift your body off the ground, keeping your wrists on the floor and your body in a straight line from head to feet.
- Engage your core muscles, including your pelvic floor, to keep your body stable.
- Hold this pose for as long as you can, aiming for 20-30 seconds to start, and steadily increasing the time as you get stronger.

B. Side Plank:
- Begin by lying on your side with your legs stacked and your arm directly under your shoulder.
- Lift your hips off the ground, keeping your body in a straight line from head to heels.

- Engage your core muscles, including your pelvic floor, to support your body.
- Hold this pose for 20-30 seconds on each side, focused on keeping your hips lifted and your body aligned.

C. Plank with Leg Lifts:
- Start in a forearm plank pose, with your arms bent and directly under your shoulders.
- Lift one leg off the ground, keeping it straight and in line with your body.
- Engage your core and pelvic floor muscles to support your body as you hold this pose.
- Hold for 10-15 seconds, then drop your leg back down and continue on the other side.
- Make sure to keep your hips level and avoid twisting or tilting your pelvis during the leg lifts.

By adding these plank variations into your workout routine, you can effectively engage your core muscles, including your pelvic floor, to improve stability and strength, leading to better control over ejaculation and improved sexual satisfaction. Start with shorter lengths and gradually increase as you build power and endurance.

3. Bridging with Leg Lifts:
Here's an easier example of bridging with leg lifts:

1. Bridge Pose:
- Lie on your back with your knees bent and feet flat
on the floor, hip-width apart.
- Press your feet into the floor as you lift your hips
towards the sky, making a straight line from your
knees to your shoulders.
- Hold this bridge pose, engaging your core and
squeezing your buttocks.

2. Leg Lifts:
- While keeping the bridge position, lift one leg off the
ground, stretching it towards the ceiling.
- Keep your hips flat and avoid bending your lower
back.
- Lower your leg back down to the starting position.
- Repeat the leg lifts on the other side.
- Continue alternate leg lifts, focusing on engaging
your pelvic floor muscles throughout the action.

By adding leg lifts to the bridge pose, you work your
hips and pelvic floor muscles simultaneously, helping
to improve strength and stability. Start with a few
repetitions on each side and gradually increase as you
get stronger.

4. Pelvic Tilts:
Here's an easier example of pelvic tilts:

1. Starting Position:
- Lie on your back on a soft surface, like a yoga mat
or couch.
- Bend your knees so that your feet are flat on the
floor, hip-width apart.

2. Pelvic Tilt:
- Take a big breath in.
- As you exhale, slowly tilt your pelvis upward towards
your belly button by pressing your lower back into the
floor.
- Engage your pelvic floor muscles as you tilt your
hips.
- Hold this pose for a few seconds, feeling the
tightness in your pelvic floor muscles.
- Inhale as you remove the tilt and return your hips to
a normal position.
- Repeat this movement for several times, focusing on
the controlled tightening and release of your pelvic
floor muscles with each tilt.

By performing pelvic tilts regularly, you can
strengthen your pelvic floor muscles and improve
pelvic alignment, which can contribute to better
control over ejaculation and improved sexual
pleasure. Start with a few repetitions and gradually
increase as you get more comfortable with the
activity.

5. Standing Hip Abduction:
Here's an easier example of standing hip abduction:

1. Starting Position:
- Stand straight with your feet hip-width apart.
- Hold onto a strong surface, like a chair or table, for
balance if needed.

2. Lift Leg to the Side:
- Shift your weight onto one leg.
- Lift the opposite leg out to the side, keeping it
straight and in line with your body.
- Keep your hips level and your core engaged to
balance your body.
- Hold this pose for a few seconds, feeling the muscles
on the side of your hip working.

3. Lower Leg:
- Slowly lower your leg back down to the starting
position.
- Repeat the action on the other side, lifting the
opposite leg out to the side.

4. Repeat:
- Alternate lifting each leg out to the side for several
times.
- Focus on keeping good balance and stability
throughout the practice.
- Keep your movements slow and controlled to
increase the activation of your hip abductor muscles.

Standing hip abduction strengthens the muscles responsible for pelvic stability and control, which can lead to better ejaculatory control and increased sexual satisfaction. Start with a few repetitions on each side and gradually increase as you get stronger.

By incorporating these exercises into your routine on a daily basis, you can strengthen your pelvic floor muscles, improve control over ejaculation, and enhance sexual pleasure. So, get ready to flex those pelvic floor muscles and take control of your sexual health and happiness!

## Chapter Five:

## Communication and Intimacy

Effective conversation and closeness are the basis of a happy and enjoyable sexual relationship. In the world of sexual intimacy, the ability to freely talk about preferences, desires, and limits with your partner can greatly improve the quality of your connection and general happiness. Moreover, fostering emotional closeness and trust lays the basis for a strong and resilient relationship. In this part, we will dig into the importance of open conversation in addressing sexual wants and desires, as well as explore methods for nurturing emotional intimacy and building trust within relationships. Through honest and respectful conversation, coupled with efforts to strengthen emotional connection, couples can foster a fulfilling and harmonious sexual relationship.

### 1. Importance of Open Communication with Partner About Sexual Preferences and Needs

Open conversation with your partner about sexual tastes and needs plays a crucial role in achieving ejaculation control and improving sexual pleasure. Here's why it's so important:

1. Understanding Each Other's Needs:
When you talk openly with your partner about what you like and what you need during sex, you both get

a better idea of what makes the other person feel good. This means you can make sex more fun for each other because you know what gets them on and what they're comfortable with. When it comes to ejaculation control, knowing each other's needs helps you figure out what works best for both of you, so you can have sex that feels amazing and lasts as long as you want it to.

2. Addressing Concerns and Challenges:
Talking frankly about any worries or troubles you might have with ejaculating too quickly, like premature ejaculation, is really important. When you share these worries with your partner, you can figure out ways to deal with them together. This might mean trying out different tricks or methods to help you last longer during sex. By talking about it, you can come up with answers that work for both of you, making your sex life more satisfying and fun.

3. Building Trust and Connection:
Sharing your deepest thoughts and feelings about what you want in bed helps build trust and a better emotional bond with your partner. When you know you can talk freely about sensitive stuff like sex without thinking about being judged, it brings you closer together. This trust makes your relationship stronger because you feel safe being yourself and sharing your wants without fear.

4. Enhancing Pleasure and Satisfaction:
Talking freely about what feels good and what you
enjoy during sex is like giving your partner a roadmap
to your happiness. When you share these things, it
helps you both have more satisfying and enjoyable
times in bed. By knowing each other's tastes, you can
try out new things or different ways of doing things
that make sex even more exciting and pleasurable.
This not only makes sex more fun, but it also helps
you both get better at controlling ejaculation and
making the experience last longer.

5. Reducing Performance Pressure:
Talking freely about your sexual preferences and
wants with your partner can actually take a lot of
pressure off both of you. When you're able to share
what you like and what you're worried about without
feeling judged, it provides a safe and relaxed
atmosphere for closeness. This means you can focus
more on enjoying each other and less on thinking
about how well you're acting. As a result, you're more
likely to feel comfortable and confident during sex,
which can help reduce the possibility of premature
ejaculation and make the experience more enjoyable
for both parties.

6. Enhancing Connection and Intimacy:
Think of open conversation as the bridge that ties you
and your partner on a deeper level. By freely sharing
your sexual preferences and wants, you bring
vulnerability and authenticity into your relationship.
This openness promotes a sense of connection and

intimacy, as you both share your deepest wants and fears without reservation. As a result, your bond gets stronger, and you feel more linked to each other both emotionally and physically.

7. Empowering Sexual Exploration:
When you and your partner talk freely about your sexual wants and needs, it's like building a strong bridge between you. This bridge helps you to connect on a deeper level, sharing your most personal thoughts and feelings without holding back. By being vulnerable and real with each other, you build a feeling of closeness and intimacy that improves your link. As you share your deepest wishes and fears, you build trust and understanding, which brings you closer together mentally and physically. This deep link improves your relationship, making you feel more connected and supported by each other, both in and out of the bedroom.

8. Cultivating Mutual Satisfaction:
When you and your partner freely discuss your sexual preferences and wants, it lays the groundwork for mutual happiness and joy in your relationship. By sharing what brings you pleasure and what you need to achieve ejaculation control, you create a collaborative sexual dynamic. This means you can work together to ensure that both of you feel deeply happy and respected in your intimate times. As you value each other's pleasure and happiness, it improves the basis of your relationship, leading to greater unity and happiness overall. Ultimately, open conversation about sexual preferences and wants is

the key to building a fulfilling and satisfying relationship where both parties feel heard, understood, and loved.

9. Tailoring Sexual Experiences:
Open conversation in your relationship allows you to customize your sexual experiences just like you would customize a music for a road trip. By freely speaking your goals and preferences, you can tailor your intimate moments to suit both you and your partner perfectly. Whether it's trying out new positions, playing with different techniques, or setting the pace for arousal, being open about what you want ensures that both partners are happy and excited about the journey ahead. Just like choosing the perfect songs for your trip, open conversation helps you create amazing moments of pleasure and connection together.

10. Overcoming Challenges Together: Ejaculation skill can sometimes come with challenges like premature ejaculation or trouble reaching climax. But with open conversation, you and your partner can face these obstacles together. By discussing these issues freely, you can work as a team to find answers. Together, you can study different strategies, try out new techniques, and help each other every step of the way. Just like navigating through a tough stretch of road on a trip, meeting these challenges together improves your bond and makes the journey to ejaculation mastery even more satisfying.

Open conversation about sexual preferences and wants lays the groundwork for achieving ejaculation mastery by supporting knowledge, confidence, and connection between partners. It allows you to address challenges, improve pleasure, and increase intimacy, eventually leading to a more fulfilling and satisfying sexual relationship.

## 2. Strategies for Fostering Emotional Intimacy and Trust in Relationships

Fostering emotional closeness and trust in partnerships is like looking at a delicate plant. Here are some strategies to foster a healthy relationship with your partner:

1. Open Communication: Just like watering your plants regularly, communication is important for nurturing mental intimacy. Talk freely and honestly with your partner about your feelings, wants, and fears. Share your ideas and experiences, and listen carefully to what your partner has to say. This provides a safe and supportive setting where trust can grow.

Let's picture your relationship is like a cozy campfire. Open conversation is the spark that keeps the fires burning bright and warm. Just as you add logs to keep the fire going, sharing your thoughts, feelings, and fears with your partner makes your bond strong and vibrant.

When you speak freely, it's like passing around a lantern in the dark. You both get to see each other's true selves, lighting up the way to understanding and trust. Whether you're sharing your dreams or talking about your fears, every chat adds fuel to the fire of emotional intimacy.

Think of open conversation as making a sturdy bridge between you and your partner. With every word you share, the bridge gets stronger, allowing you to cross over to each other's hearts with ease. This bridge of conversation is what holds your relationship together, even during bad weather.

So, keep the lines of communication open like a clear night sky full of stars. Share your hopes, dreams, and even your silly jokes. As you do, you'll find that your bond with your partner gets deeper and stronger, producing a love that shines brighter than any fire in the night.

2. Vulnerability:  Just as sunshine nourishes your yard, vulnerability is the light that supports emotional closeness. Be ready to show your real self to your partner, including your strengths and weaknesses. Share your hopes and dreams, as well as your fears and doubts. When you both feel comfortable being vulnerable with each other, it improves your relationship and strengthens your bond.

Imagine weakness as a magic potion in your relationship, a potion that brings you and your partner closer together than ever before. It's like opening up a treasure chest full of secret gems – your inner thoughts, fears, and dreams.

When you're open with your partner, it's like taking off your shield and showing them your true self. You let them see your quirks, your flaws, and your weaknesses, knowing that they'll accept you just as you are. This forms a special link between you, like two puzzle pieces fitting perfectly together.

Think of weakness as putting seeds in a garden. Each seed represents a little piece of your heart that you share with your partner. As you water these seeds with honesty and trust, they grow into beautiful flowers of emotional connection, filling your relationship with love and joy.

Being vulnerable is like opening the door to your inner world and asking your partner in for a nice chat by the fireplace. You share your hopes and dreams, your fears and worries, knowing that they'll hold your hand and walk with you through it all. This strengthens your relationship and builds a foundation of trust that's as solid as a rock.

So, don't be afraid to be open with your partner. Embrace it like a secret gift that strengthens your bond and makes your love shine brighter than ever before.

3. Empathy: Like fertilizer improves the earth, empathy nourishes your relationship. Put yourself in your partner's shoes and try to understand their view. Show sympathy and understanding towards their feelings and experiences, even if you don't always agree. This cultivates a sense of understanding and support, promoting emotional closeness and trust.

Imagine empathy as a magical mirror in your relationship, mirroring back the thoughts and emotions of your partner. It's like stepping into their shoes and seeing the world through their eyes, understanding their joys and pains as if they were your own.

When you practice understanding with your partner, it's like sending out a gentle breeze on a hot day. Your empathy cools their worries and soothes their fears, creating a safe and comfortable place where they feel truly understood and cared for.

Think of empathy as a warm hug on a cold day. When your partner is feeling down or stressed, your empathy wraps around them like a cozy blanket, letting them know that they're not alone in their challenges. This improves your bond and builds trust, knowing that you'll always be there for each other no matter what.

Being empathetic is like being a detective, looking for hints to your partner's thoughts and emotions. You listen with your heart, picking up on their subtle cues and nuances, and reacting with kindness and understanding. This strengthens your relationship and creates a sense of intimacy that's as comforting as a known song.

So, learn to understand your partner every day. Let them know that you're there for them, ready to listen and support them in any way you can. As you do, you'll find that your relationship blossoms and thrives, getting stronger and more beautiful with each passing day.

4. Quality Time: Just as trees need time to grow, relationships require quality time together to blossom. Make an effort to spend valuable time with your partner, free from distractions and responsibilities. Engage in activities you both enjoy, whether it's going for a walk, cooking together, or simply sitting on the couch. This concentrated time strengthens your relationship and builds mental intimacy.

Imagine quality time as a treasure box in your relationship, filled with valuable moments and treasured memories. It's like going on a grand journey with your partner, exploring new places and finding hidden gems along the way.

When you spend valuable time together, it's like planting seeds in a yard. Each moment you share is like watering those seeds, nurturing your bond and making it grow stronger and more lively with each passing day.

Think of leisure time as a cozy dinner in the park. You spread out a blanket, unpack a delicious feast, and spend hours laughing, talking, and simply enjoying each other's company. It's these easy times of togetherness that build a strong base of trust and intimacy in your relationship.

Quality time is like a warm hug on a cold day. It wraps you and your partner in a blanket of love and affection, providing a safe and comforting place where you can be yourselves without any pretenses or masks.

So, make time for each other regularly, whether it's a romantic dinner date, a relaxed walk in the park, or a cozy night in watching movies. As you do, you'll find that your relationship blooms and grows, becoming a source of joy, comfort, and strength for both of you.

5. Affection and Praise: Like flowers grow with gentle care, affection and praise strengthen your relationship. Show your partner love and affection through physical touch, kind words, and acts of gratitude. Express thanks for the little things they do, and let them know how much you value them. This promotes a sense of comfort and connection, deepening your emotional link.

Imagine love and praise as the sunshine and rain in your relationship garden. Affection is like the warm rays of the sun, while respect is like the gentle rain that nourishes the land.

Affection is like spreading magic dust on your bond. It's the little actions – a hug, a kiss, a loving touch – that make your partner feel treasured and appreciated. It's these small acts of kindness that build a strong base of love and trust.

Appreciation is like watering your relationship garden with thanks. It's taking the time to notice and praise the things your partner does for you, big and small. Whether it's a kind word, a thoughtful act, or simply being there for you when you need them, expressing thanks strengthens your bond and deepens your relationship.

Together, affection and recognition produce a beautiful garden of love and trust. They nurture your relationship, helping it grow and thrive even in the toughest times. So, don't forget to shower your partner with love and praise every day. As you do, you'll find that your relationship grows and blooms, becoming more beautiful and strong with each passing day.

6. Shared Goals and Values: Just as a plant needs a common vision, shared goals and values connect you and your partner. Discuss your goals, dreams, and beliefs, and find common ground to build upon. Work together towards agreed goals, helping each other along the way. This shared sense of purpose improves your relationship and promotes emotional closeness.

Imagine shared goals and values as the guide leading your relationship journey. It's like setting sail on a big trip together, knowing that you're going in the same direction and navigating through life's ups and downs as a team.

Shared goals are like planting seeds in your relationship yard. They're the dreams and goals you both hold dear, whether it's getting a home, starting a family, or traveling the world. By working towards these goals together, you improve your bond and build a sense of unity and purpose in your relationship.

Shared beliefs are like the bricks that make the basis of your connection. They're the values and views you both hold dear, such as honesty, loyalty, and respect. When your beliefs align, it provides a solid framework of trust and understanding, allowing you to weather any storm that comes your way.

Together, shared goals and values form a plan for your relationship journey. They provide direction and meaning, leading you through life's twists and turns with confidence and clarity. So, take the time to discover your shared goals and beliefs with your partner. As you do, you'll find that your relationship gets stronger and more resilient, forming a bond that's as unbreakable as it is beautiful.

7. Active Listening: Active listening is like setting seeds of understanding in the garden of your

connection. It's about giving your partner your full attention, like watering your plants with care and attention. When you actively listen, you're not just hearing your partner's words – you're truly tuning in to their thoughts and emotions, nurturing a stronger bond between you.

Imagine active hearing as a dance between two partners, moving in perfect rhythm. You take turns leading and following, imitating each other's moves with grace and understanding. By hearing carefully and reacting with empathy and understanding, you create a safe and helpful place where both partners feel valued and appreciated.

So, next time your partner talks, imagine yourself tending to a delicate flower in your relationship yard. Listen with your heart, nurture their words with care, and watch as your bond blooms and flourishes with each moment of real connection.

8. Respect and Support: Respect and support are like the sturdy walls keeping up the roof of your relationship home. They provide stability and power, providing a safe and secure place where love can flourish and grow.

Imagine respect as the golden rule in your relationship garden. Just as you would treat yourself with kindness and respect, so too should you treat your partner. Respect their views, beliefs, and limits, and respect their individuality and autonomy. By doing so, you foster a culture of mutual respect and understanding, where both partners feel respected and appreciated.

Support is like the safety net beneath a tightrope walker, ready to catch them if they fall. It's about being there for your partner through thick and thin, giving a listening ear, a helping hand, or a shoulder to lean on when they need it most. Whether it's enjoying their successes or comforting them in times of sadness, your unwavering support strengthens your bond and increases your connection.

So, tend to the pillars of love and support in your relationship garden with care and purpose. Water them with kindness, nurture them with understanding, and watch as they grow stronger and more resilient with each passing day, giving a solid base for love to thrive.

9. Forgiveness and Growth: Forgiveness and growth are like the sunshine and rain in your relationship garden. They nourish and rejuvenate, promoting new starts and fresh views.

Imagine forgiveness as the gentle rain that washes away the past, allowing new seeds of love to take root and blossom. It's about letting go of anger and grudges, and opening your heart to healing and forgiveness. By forgiving your partner's mistakes and shortcomings, you make room for growth and rebirth in your partnership.

Growth is like the warm rays of the sun, illuminating the way forward and encouraging new options. It's about accepting obstacles and setbacks as chances for learning and growth, both personally and as a couple. By committing to personal growth and development, you support a relationship that's constantly evolving and thriving.

So, tend to the garden of forgiveness and progress in your relationship with care and purpose. Water it with forgiveness, allowing old scars to heal and new starts to bloom. And nourish it with growth, accepting each challenge as a chance for change and renewal. As you do, you'll watch your relationship garden thrive and bloom with energy and resilience.

10. Shared Vulnerabilities: Shared vulnerabilities are like setting seeds of trust and closeness in the fertile soil of your relationship. It's about being strong enough to show your tender roots and delicate petals, knowing that your partner will foster and protect them with care.

Imagine sharing weaknesses as opening up the seed packet of your heart and pouring its contents into the land of your connection. You share your fears, doubts, and past experiences, allowing them to take root and grow alongside your partner's. Together, you tend to these seeds with love and understanding, watering them with kindness and acceptance.

As these seeds of vulnerability sprout and grow, they build a tapestry of trust and closeness between you and your partner. You create a safe place where you can be your true selves, free from criticism or shame. By sharing vulnerabilities, you strengthen your emotional link and foster a relationship that is strong, resilient, and deeply based in love.

So, accept the beauty of shared weaknesses in your relationship garden. Plant seeds of trust and closeness with courage and openness, and watch as they bloom into a beautiful garden of love and understanding, where you and your partner can flourish together.

By nurturing these tactics, you can create a thriving garden of emotional closeness and trust that continues to bloom and thrive over time. Just as with gardening, it takes patience, dedication, and nurturing care, but the benefits are well worth the effort.

# Chapter Six:

## Behavioral Techniques

Welcome to the world of behavioral techniques – your toolbox for mastering ejaculation and improving sexual pleasure. Just like a skilled cook carefully chooses the right ingredients to create a masterpiece, these techniques empower you to take control of your arousal and prolong the pleasure of intimacy.

In this chapter, we'll explore real strategies for managing arousal and slowing ejaculation, from simple distraction techniques to creative changes in sexual positions. Get ready to open the secrets to a fulfilling and enduring sexual experience, where you can enjoy every moment and take your pleasure to new heights. Let's dive in and learn the art of ejaculation skill together!

### 1. Behavioral Strategies for Managing Arousal and Delaying Ejaculation.

Managing arousal and delaying ejaculation is like leading a concert of feelings, where you are the master directing each note to create a harmonious and satisfying experience. Let's delve into the behavioral tactics that can help you learn this art and prolong the pleasure of intimacy:

1. Sensory Control:
Sensory control is like changing the volume knob on
your favorite song – you have the power to dial up or
dial down the intensity of feeling during sexual action.
Start by exploring different touches, forces, and
moves to see what feels good and what helps you
stay in control. If you feel like you're getting too close
to climax, take a break or switch to a softer touch
until you're ready to continue. It's all about finding
the right mix of excitement to keep arousal at a
steady simmer without boiling over too soon.

2. Breathing Techniques:
Breathing techniques are like taking deep breaths to
calm down before a big moment. Start by breathing
slowly through your nose, filling your belly with air.
Hold it for a moment, then exhale slowly through your
mouth, relaxing stress as you breathe out. Focus on
keeping your breath deep and steady, syncing it with
your moves to stay relaxed and in control during
intimate times.

3. Mindfulness and Distraction:
Mindfulness and distraction are like changing the
station on your TV to stay focused during a movie.
With mindfulness, you stay present in the moment by
paying attention to what's happening right now, like
the feelings in your body or the things around you. If
your mind starts to wander towards climax, slowly
bring it back to the present moment. Distraction is
like hitting pause on those thoughts by giving your
brain something else to focus on, like counting or

looking at an object in the room. It helps shift your mind away from excitement so you can stay in control.

4. Change of Pace and Position:
Changing pace and position is like changing the speed and style of your dance moves to keep the party going. Try out different positions that offer a bit less excitement or give you more control over your desire. Mix it up with slow and steady moves, then add in some faster-paced action to keep things interesting. By switching things up, you can lengthen the fun without running to the finish line.

5. Pelvic Floor Exercises:
Pelvic floor exercises are like training lessons for the muscles that help you stay in control during the big event. Just like lifting weights improves your arms, kegel exercises and other pelvic floor workouts build those important muscles down below. Practice squeezing and releasing them during private moments to build up your control and lengthen the pleasure. It's like having a strong foundation to back you through the whole show.

6. Communication and Partner Collaboration:
Communication and collaboration with your partner are like having a trusted friend by your side during a game. By freely talking about what you both want and need, you can create a game plan to handle arousal and make the most of your time together. Share your thoughts, listen to your partner's opinion, and brainstorm ideas to keep the excitement going. With

teamwork and understanding, you can handle the challenges of ejaculation control together and score big in the joy department.

7. Sensate Focus:

Sensate focus is like fine-tuning your instrument before the big show—it helps you and your partner get in sync and explore each other's bodies without thinking about the grand finish. Take turns touching and exploring, focused on the pleasure of the moment rather than hitting the finish line. This exercise improves your bond and extends the excitement, making the experience more rewarding for both of you.

8. Visualization and Mental Imagery:

Visualization is like making a thought movie where you're the star of the show. Close your eyes and picture yourself in a peaceful, stress-free setting, where you're in full control of your desire. Visualize yourself staying longer and feeling confident in your skills. By drawing this picture in your mind, you can rewire your thinking and improve your ability to control ejaculation, leading to a more satisfying experience for you and your partner.

9. Scheduled Ejaculation:

Scheduled ejaculation is like penciling in time for practice lessons in your busy schedule. Set aside specific moments with your partner where you focus on slowing ejaculation. By consciously holding back during these workouts, you can gradually train your body to last longer. Think of it as building up your energy for the main event, helping you stay in control and prolong pleasure when it counts.

10. Self-awareness and Reflection:
Self-awareness and thought are like having a backstage pass to your own show. Take moments to think on your sexual encounters, noting what factors may influence your desire and ejaculation. Keep a journal to track trends, triggers, and the usefulness of different methods. By knowing yourself better, you can fine-tune your approach to ejaculation skill, ensuring a more satisfying performance each time.

By adding these behavioral tactics into your sexual routine, you can develop greater control over your arousal and ejaculation reaction. Remember that ejaculation mastery is a trip, not a goal, and it may take time and practice to find what works best for you and your partner. Stay curious, stay open-minded, and enjoy the process of discovering new ways to improve your sexual satisfaction and intimacy.

## 2. Distraction Techniques and Changing Sexual Positions to Prolong Intercourse

1. Distraction Techniques:
Engage in light distraction: When you feel arousal growing too quickly, shift your focus away from sexual feelings by thinking about something non-sexual or mundane. Counting backward from 100 or reciting the words of your favorite song can shift your attention and help delay ejaculation.

Practice mindfulness: Stay present in the moment by focusing on your feelings and the physical experiences of closeness. Notice the touch of your partner's skin, the sound of their breathing, and the warmth of their body against yours. Mindfulness can help avoid unwanted thinking about climax and lengthen arousal.

Let's dig deeper into distraction methods to prolong intercourse:

1. Sensory Distraction:
Engage in sensory activities: Incorporate sensory experiences into your sexual encounters to shift attention away from desire. Try adding sense exercises to your intimacy: Introduce new feelings during lovemaking to change attention away from desire. For example, you could use ice cubes or feathers to produce tingling feelings on your partner's skin, helping to separate from strong arousal and lengthen the experience.

2. Cognitive Distraction:
Play mental games: Challenge your mind by playing games or solving problems with your partner during closeness. This helps redirect attention from sexual feelings, giving you more control over arousal and prolonging the experience. Play word association games, answer riddles or tasks together, or engage in light-hearted talk about non-sexual topics to move attention away from arousal.

3. Physical Distraction:
Switch focus: Instead of simply focusing on genital stimulation, explore other areas of your partner's body during heightened desire. Kiss, caress, or rub parts like the neck, shoulders, or back to introduce pleasant distractions, extending the private experience and delaying ejaculation.

4. Environmental Distraction:
Change the surroundings: Shake things up by changing where you have sex.  Change the setting of your sexual encounters to introduce new triggers that catch your attention.

Try different locations like the bedroom, living room, or even outdoors to introduce fresh sensations that can shift your focus, adding excitement and prolonging intercourse.

5. Self-Talk and Visualization:
Positive reinforcement: Harness the power of self-talk and visualization to boost your confidence in controlling ejaculation. Repeat affirmations such as "I have control over my arousal" or "I can prolong ejaculation" to promote an attitude of confidence and power. Visualize yourself successfully delaying ejaculation, focused on the feelings and emotions linked with delayed pleasure.

6. Focused Breathing:
Deep breathing techniques: Employ focused breathing exercises to soothe the nervous system and shift attention away from strong excitement. Inhale deeply through your nose, hold for a short moment, and release slowly through your mouth. This intentional breathing pattern promotes calm, helping to delay ejaculation and prolong intimacy.

7. Role-Playing and Fantasy:
Embrace role-playing scenarios or dig into shared dreams to transport yourselves into an alternate story, diverting attention from approaching ejaculation. Experiment with various parts, outfits, or scenarios to spark imagination and extend arousal, allowing for a longer and more satisfying personal experience.

8. Multi-Sensory Experiences:
Infuse your personal moments with multi-sensory experiences to overload the senses and draw attention away from excitement. Set the scene with relaxing music, fragrant candles, or soft lighting to create an ambiance that amplifies pleasure while offering a diversion from the rush of ejaculation.

9. Humor and Playfulness:
Inject humor and playfulness into your lovemaking to ease stress and reduce performance anxiety. Share jokes, engage in lighthearted banter, or partake in playful tickling or fighting to promote laughs and shift attention from the pressure of ejaculation.

10. Mindfulness and Grounding Techniques: Embrace
mindfulness and grounding practices to tether
yourself to the present and prevent intrusive thoughts
or worries from stopping arousal. Tune into your
feelings, like the sensation of touch or the sound of
your partner's words, to stay grounded and tied to the
moment.

11. Utilize Props or Sex Toys:
Integrate props or sex toys into your sexual routine to
introduce fresh feelings and diversions. Experiment
with items like vibrators, blindfolds, or restraints to
add excitement and variation, thus increasing
pleasure.

12. Engage in Foreplay:
Invest in ample foreplay to heighten anticipation and
extend libido prior to intercourse. Explore various
erogenous zones, indulge in intense kissing, or join in
mutual masturbation to increase arousal and
postpone ejaculation.

By incorporating these distraction methods into your
sexual encounters, you and your partner can prolong
intercourse and improve happiness while learning
ejaculation control. Experiment with different
techniques to discover what works best for you and
your partner's wants and tastes.

2. Changing Sexual Positions
Slow and Steady: Opt for sexual positions that allow
for slower, more controlled movements, lowering the
strength of stimulation and prolonging desire.
Positions like missionary with the woman's legs closed
or spooning provide less pressure and may help delay
ejaculation.

Experiment with Angles: Explore sexual positions that
reduce insertion depth or change the angle of
penetration to lower sensitivity and prolong
intercourse. Positions like cowgirl or reverse cowgirl
allow the receiving partner to control the pace and
depth of penetration, allowing opportunities to change
stimulation levels.

Incorporate Breaks: Intersperse moments of rest or
non-penetrative closeness between position changes
to give both partners a chance to cool down and
increase the overall length of intercourse.

Here are more tips on changing sexual positions to
continue intercourse:

1. Variety and Exploration: Try out different sexual
situations with your partner to find ones that work
best for both of you. Experiment with various angles,
depths, and levels of entry to discover what feels
most enjoyable and helps you last longer before
reaching pleasure.

2. Strategic Position Selection: Pick sexual poses that naturally lessen stimulation to the penis or offer better control over arousal. Positions like spooning or side-by-side allow for deeper penetration, lowering excitement and helping to lengthen intercourse.

3. Communication and Collaboration: Talk freely with your partner about which sexual positions help you last longer during intercourse. Work together to try out different positions and share comments on what works best for both of you..

4. Incorporate Rest and Pause: Build breaks into your lovemaking by switching between sexual poses. Transitioning gives you short times to catch your breath and regulate arousal, helping to extend the length of intercourse.

5. Focus on Mutual Pleasure: Embrace sexual situations that value mutual pleasure and closeness, ensuring both parties can fully engage in the experience without solely focused on ejaculation control. Positions like joint stimulation or oral sex provide different routes for pleasure while helping to delay ejaculation.

6. Experiment with Control Techniques: Try out sexual situations that allow for control techniques like pacing, changing thrusting patterns, or different rhythms. By fine-tuning the speed and intensity of intercourse according to arousal levels, you can successfully delay

ejaculation while ensuring optimal pleasure for both parties.

7. Utilize Supportive Props: Incorporate supportive props or furniture like pillows, cushions, or sex wedges to improve comfort and stability during various sexual poses. These props offer extra support and leverage, allowing longer-lasting intercourse without pain or tiredness.

8. Embrace Sensual Connection: Prioritize keeping a deep sense of sensual connection and closeness with your partner, independent of the sexual position. Emphasize eye contact, verbal conversation, and physical touch to improve mental connection and extend the total experience of closeness.

9. Utilize Transitional Positions: Integrate transitional sexual positions that offer moments of ease while moving between more exciting ones. For instance, moving from a highly stimulating position to one with less energy provides short breaks to control arousal levels and extend intercourse.

10. Focus on External Stimulation: Try sexual poses that stress external stimulation of erogenous zones like the clitoris, perineum, or nipples. By directing attention to external pleasure, you can lessen penile stimulation strength, prolong intercourse, and keep mutual happiness.

11. Alternate Between Active and Passive Roles:
Switch between situations where one person is more
active in moving and stimulation, while the other
takes a passive role. This alternation allows for times
of both heightened arousal and rest, helping in
controlling arousal levels and extending intercourse.

12. Integrate Sensory Deprivation Techniques:
Experiment with sensory deprivation methods like
blindfolding or using earplugs to heighten non-genital
sensations and lower focus on sexual stimulus. This
can lengthen arousal, delay ejaculation, and improve
total sexual pleasure and intimacy.

13. Create a Playful Atmosphere: Infuse your sexual
meetings with a playful and spontaneous vibe by
bringing elements of fun and laughs. Try unusual
positions or role-playing scenarios to keep things
light-hearted and engaged, prolonging arousal and
happiness.

14. Customize Positions to Fit Your Bodies: Tailor
sexual positions to fit the specific anatomy and tastes
of both partners. Make changes in angles, depths, or
variations of positions to best comfort, pleasure, and
control over arousal. This ensures a pleasurable and
satisfactory experience tailored to each individual's
wants.

15. Prioritize Emotional Connection: Make emotional connection the main point of your sexual action with your partner. Emphasize strengthening your bond, showing love and respect, and promoting mutual trust and understanding. By valuing emotional connection, you create a helpful and nurturing setting that supports prolonged intercourse and ejaculation control.

By incorporating these tactics and experiencing a diverse range of sexual positions, you and your partner can prolong intercourse, improve satisfaction, and master ejaculation control together. Remember to speak openly, value mutual pleasure, and welcome experimentation to discover what works best for your unique preferences and wants.

Remember, conversation with your partner is key when exploring distraction methods and changing sexual positions. Be open to trying new things together and giving comments to ensure a mutually satisfying experience.

# Chapter Seven:

## Delay Tactics

Welcome to the land of sexual mastery, where the art of delaying climax turns everyday moments into extraordinary experiences. In this part, we start on a trip through the world of close connection, exploring tactics and techniques meant to prolong pleasure and raise happiness. From classic moves like the stop-start and squeeze methods to novel approaches, we'll unravel the secrets to achieving greater control over your sexual reaction. So, prepare to start on an adventure of discovery, where each tactic becomes a tool in your arsenal for improving intimacy and strengthening your connection with your partner.

## 1. Specific Tactics and Techniques for Delaying Climax During Sexual Activity

Let's start on a trip into the land of delaying climax during private moments, where each tactic becomes a key to releasing prolonged pleasure. Imagine yourself as an explorer, navigating the complex world of sexual feelings with interest and skill. Here, we'll dive into specific techniques meant to extend the journey of arousal and elevate the experience of intimacy.

1. The Stop-Start Method:
Picture yourself as a skilled musician, directing the beat of arousal with precision. With the stop-start

method, you'll learn to pause and restart sexual action carefully, allowing arousal to ebb and flow like the tide. By learning this method, you gain the power to prolong the trip towards climax, savoring each moment of heightened feeling.

The stop-start method is like pressing the pause button during sexual action to prevent reaching orgasm too fast. When you feel yourself getting too close to climax, you or your partner pause all stimulation for a moment or switch to a less exciting activity. This break allows the arousal to drop slightly, giving you more control over when you finish. Once you feel ready, you can restart sexual action at a slower pace or with less strong stimulation. It's like taking breaks during a run to catch your breath and pace yourself, ensuring you can go the route without finishing too soon.

2. The Squeeze Technique:
Imagine yourself as a sculptor, shaping the strength of desire with care. With the squeeze method, you'll learn to apply gentle pressure to the base of the penis to briefly halt ejaculation. Like shaping clay, you can shape the experience of pleasure, stalling climax while keeping a steady pace of arousal.

The squeeze method involves giving gentle pressure to the base of the penis just before reaching the point of climax. This pressure helps to temporarily lower erection and delay ejaculation. It's like putting your foot on the brakes to slow down a moving car. When you or your partner feels like ejaculation is close, you gently squeeze the base of the penis for a few seconds until the urge to ejaculate fades. This interruption allows you to recover control over your arousal levels and continue sexual activity. It's a bit like hitting the pause button during a movie to take a breather before jumping back in.

3. Breathing and Relaxation:
Envision yourself as a master of the breath, mastering its power to regulate excitement. Through deep breathing and relaxation methods, you'll learn to calm the nervous system and control the intensity of feeling. By syncing your breath with each movement, you create a rhythm of pleasure that extends the journey towards climax, allowing for greater connection and satisfaction.

Breathing and calming methods are like the conductor's baton, directing the music of arousal with ease and accuracy. By learning deep breathing, you tap into the body's natural ability to calm the nervous system and reduce stress. With each inhale, you draw in rest and calm, while each exhale releases any pent-up tension or worry. Syncing your breath with sexual moves produces a harmonious beat, prolonging the rise of arousal and delays climax. It's like riding the waves of pleasure, allowing you to savor each moment and strengthen the bond with your partner. As you become more attuned to your breath and body, you gain greater control over your arousal levels, improving closeness and happiness.

4. Mental Distraction:
Picture yourself as a magician, creating tricks of distraction to captivate the mind. By engaging in mental activities or moving focus to non-sexual thoughts, you can distract attention away from approaching climax. Like a magician's sleight of hand, these distractions create times of pause, stretching the experience of pleasure and intimacy.

Mental distraction methods are similar to the magician's art, where the mind becomes the stage for redirecting attention away from climax. Engaging in mental activities or focusing on non-sexual thoughts causes a brief break in the intensity of desire, similar to pulling a rabbit out of a hat. By shifting your focus to chores like solving puzzles or remembering a favorite memory, you create a mental world where arousal takes a back seat. This brief diversion allows arousal to plateau, lengthening the journey towards climax and improving total pleasure. Just as a magician captivates their audience with illusions, mental distraction methods captivate the mind, extending the pleasure of intimacy with your partner.

5. Communication and Collaboration:
See yourself as a collaborator, working hand in hand with your partner to lengthen the experience of pleasure. By freely talking desires, tastes, and tactics for delaying climax, you build a shared understanding that improves intimacy. Through teamwork, you discover new options for pleasure, improving the journey of sexual exploration.

Communication and teamwork in delaying climax is like being part of a team, where you and your partner work together towards a shared goal of prolonging pleasure. It's about freely talking with each other about what you both enjoy and what techniques work best to delay climax. By sharing your thoughts, tastes, and ideas, you build a better connection and understanding, making the experience more intimate and satisfying. Together, you explore new ways to prolong pleasure and strengthen your bond, changing your sexual encounters into a collaborative adventure.

6. Sensate Focus:
Imagine yourself as a director of feelings, arranging a symphony of touch and pleasure. With sensate focus, you and your partner start on a journey of discovery, finding new paths to arousal and delaying climax. By focusing on the physical experience rather than the end goal, you can lengthen the moments of closeness, strengthening your connection and pleasure.

Sensate focus is like being an explorer of touch and pleasure, traveling through a world of feelings with your partner. Instead of running towards climax, you take your time to explore each other's bodies, focused on how different touches feel and how they make you both feel. It's about enjoying the trip of intimacy, prolonging the times of pleasure, and strengthening your bond with your partner. By prioritizing sensory experiences over hitting the finish line, you build a more rewarding and satisfying sexual relationship.

7. Role-Playing and Fantasy:
See yourself as a storyteller, weaving tales of dream
and desire to lengthen the excitement of sexual
interactions. Through role-playing scenarios and
shared dreams, you build a world of adventure and
intrigue where time seems to stand still. By
immersing yourselves in these tales, you can extend
the length of arousal, sparking desire and
expectation.

Role-playing and imagination are like going into a
world of make-believe, where you and your partner
can become anyone you want to be. Whether you're
playing out a secret dream or imagining yourselves in
a different setting, the key is to let your mind run
wild. By getting lost in these role-playing scenarios,
you can extend the excitement and expectation,
making every moment feel like an adventure. It's
about discovering new characters and scenes
together, keeping the passion alive and the arousal
levels high.

8. Physical Techniques:
Envision yourself as a master of your own body,
utilizing physical techniques to delay climax and
lengthen pleasure. Techniques such as the pelvic floor
movements, where you strengthen and control your
pelvic muscles, give you the power to manage arousal
and lengthen the trip towards climax. By mastering
these methods, you improve your ability to maintain
arousal and satisfaction.

Physical methods are like discovering the secrets of your body's own control panel. With exercises like pelvic floor movements, you're improving the muscles that play a crucial role in arousal and ejaculation. It's like having a secret tool in your arsenal, giving you the ability to control arousal levels and increase pleasure. By learning these physical methods, you gain greater control over your body's reactions, leading to a more satisfying and prolonged sexual experience.

9. Exploration of Erotic Zones:
Picture yourself as an adventurer, exploring the unexplored regions of your partner's body. By finding and stimulating erogenous zones beyond the genitals, you can stretch arousal and delay climax. Explore areas such as the neck, ears, and inner thighs, where touch sparks a fire of desire that feeds prolonged closeness.

Exploring erotic zones is like going on a thrilling journey, finding secret treasures of pleasure in your partner's body. Imagine tracing the curves of their neck, teasing their ears, or kissing their inner legs – each touch sparking a spark of desire that prolongs arousal. By going beyond the obvious, you open up new paths to pleasure, extending the journey towards climax and deepening intimacy between you and your partner.

10. Creative Foreplay:
See yourself as an artist, creating lines of anticipation and desire through creative foreplay. Experiment with

different methods and activities, such as sensual massages, fun teasing, or sexual stories, to build arousal gradually and delay climax. By engaging in these artistic expressions of desire, you lengthen the trip of closeness and strengthen the connection with your partner.

In this world of delayed satisfaction, each tactic becomes a brushstroke on the canvas of intimacy, drawing a picture of connection and joy. So, accept your role as an explorer of happiness, and start on this trip with curiosity, imagination, and an open heart.

## 2. Instruction on Some Effective Delay Tactics

Let's break down the step-by-step directions for each delay tactic:

1. The Stop-Start Method:

Step 1: Start Slowly: Begin sexual action as normal, whether it's intercourse or other forms of arousal.

Step 2: Pause at the Right Moment: As you feel yourself nearing ejaculation, pause or stop all sexual action totally.

Step 3: Relax and Regroup: Take this pause as a chance to relax your muscles and focus on managing your desire. You can use deep breathing or other calming methods here.

Step 4: Resume with Caution: Once you feel more in control, slowly resume sexual action. Start with gentle stimulation and gradually increase strength as you feel relaxed.

Step 5: Repeat as Needed: If you feel yourself nearing ejaculation again, repeat the process by stopping and gathering before continuing.

Additional ideas for the Stop-Start Method:
Timing is Key: Pay close attention to your body's signals and pause sexual action before hitting the point of no return. Learning to notice your arousal levels and intervening early can help you master this method.

Use Communication: Don't hesitate to talk with your partner about adopting the stop-start method. They can provide support and understanding, making it easier to pause and restart sexual behavior as needed.

Practice Makes Perfect: Like any skill, learning the stop-start method takes practice. Don't get frustrated if it doesn't work perfectly the first time. Keep experimenting and improving your skill over time.
2. The Squeeze Technique:
Step 1: Begin Sexual Activity: Like with the stop-start method, start sexual activity as normal.

Step 2: Identify the Right Moment: When you feel ejaculation is near, either you or your partner gently squeezes the base of the penis, just below the head.

Step 3: Hold the Squeeze: Maintain the pressure for a few seconds until the urge to ejaculate stops.

Step 4: Release and Resume: After the squeeze, release the pressure and continue with sexual action. Take it slow at first, then gradually increase pressure as desired.

Step 5: Practice Makes Perfect: With practice, you'll learn to find the right time for the squeeze and how much pressure to apply to effectively delay ejaculation.

Additional ideas for the Squeeze Technique:
Find the Right Pressure: Experiment with different amounts of pressure when performing the push. Too much pressure may be uncomfortable, while too little may not properly prevent ejaculation. Find the sweet spot that works best for you.

Involve Your Partner: If you're using the squeeze method, talk with your partner about when to apply pressure and how much. They can provide feedback and adjust their method properly to maximize success.
Combine with Other Techniques: The squeeze method can be combined with other delay tactics, such as breathing and relaxation, for improved efficiency.

Don't hesitate to try with different combos to find what works best for you.

3. Breathing and Relaxation:

Step 1: Focus on Your Breath: During physical action, pay attention to your breathing. Take slow, deep breaths in through your nose and out through your mouth.

Step 2: Relax Your Muscles: Consciously relax your pelvic muscles and any other tight places in your body. Imagine releasing stress with each breath.

Step 3: Stay Present: Use mindfulness methods to stay present in the moment and keep your mind from wandering to thoughts of climax.

Step 4: Control Your beat: Sync your breathing with the beat of sexual action, keeping a steady pace to prolong arousal without rushing towards ejaculation.

Step 5: Enjoy the Experience: By focusing on your breath and rest, you can extend the pleasure of closeness and delay ejaculation naturally.
Additional ideas for Breathing and Relaxation methods:
Practice Outside of Sexual Activity: Incorporate deep breathing and calming practices into your daily routine, not just during sexual activity. This can help you build the skills and habits needed to effectively control excitement in the moment.

Focus on Sensations: Use your breath as a tool to stay grounded in your body and present in the moment. Pay attention to the physical feelings of touch and pleasure, allowing yourself to fully experience each moment without rushing towards climax.

Stay Patient: Learning to control tension through breathing and calmness takes time and patience. Be kind to yourself and enjoy small wins along the way. With constant practice, you'll gradually build greater control over your arousal levels.

4. Mental Distraction:

Step 1: Shift Your Focus: When you feel desire rising, actively shift your attention away from sexual feelings to something non-sexual.

Step 2: Engage in a Mental Task: Try engaging in mental activities like counting backwards from 100, reciting the alphabet backward, or working easy math problems in your head.

Step 3: Visualize Calming Scenes: Picture yourself in a peaceful, relaxing setting, such as a beach or a quiet forest. Imagine the sights, sounds, and feelings of this scene to distract from desire.
Step 4: Stay Engaged: Keep your mind busy with the mental job or visualization until the urge to ejaculate subsides.

Step 5: Return to the Moment: Once you feel more in control, refocus your mind on the present moment and continue with sexual action.

Additional ideas for Mental Distraction methods: Practice Mindfulness: Incorporate mindfulness meditation into your daily routine to improve your ability to shift attention away from sexual desire. Focus on the present moment and watch thoughts without judgment, letting them pass without getting caught up in them.

Involve in Hobbies: Find activities that fully involve your mind and provide a mental break from sexual thoughts. Whether it's reading, cooking, or playing music, immerse yourself in activities that bring you joy and success outside of the bedroom.

Be Patient with Yourself: It's normal for confusing thoughts to still emerge despite your efforts. Instead of getting upset, gently guide your attention back to the present moment and continue with the chosen distraction method. Over time, you'll become more skilled at redirecting your attention.

5. Sensory Control:

Step 1: Gather Sensory Items: Collect different things such as feathers, ice cubes, silk scarves, or massage oils to create a sensory experience during sexual action.

Step 2: Experiment with Sensations: Begin by discovering different feelings on your partner's body. Use the things you've gathered to gently trigger different areas, paying attention to their emotions and preferences.

Step 3: Alternate Between Sensations: Alternate between warm and cool feelings to provide contrast and lengthen pleasure. Experiment with temperature play by using warm massage oils or ice cubes, changing the strength based on your

Step 4: Communication and Feedback: Throughout the process, talk with your partner about what feels pleasant and what feelings they enjoy most. Encourage open conversation and provide feedback to ensure the experience is enjoyable

Additional ideas for the Sensory Control method: Experiment with feelings: Explore different feelings and textures during sexual action to escape from excessive arousal. Use items like feathers, ice cubes, or silk scarves to gently stimulate different parts of the body, moving attention away from impending climax.
Temperature Play: Incorporate temperature play by switching between warm and cool feelings.
Experiment with hot wax, ice packs, or warm massage oils to create contrasting feelings on the skin, increasing excitement and slowing ejaculation.

6. Edging Technique:

Step 1: Stimulate to Near Climax: Begin by exciting yourself or your partner until you're close to orgasm. Use methods such as oral sex, manual stimulation, or penetration to build desire gradually.

Step 2: Pause or Decrease Stimulation: Once you or your partner is nearing climax, pause or decrease stimulation to avoid ejaculation. Focus on calming methods such as deep breathing to keep arousal without reaching orgasm.

Step 3: Repeat the Cycle: Repeat the cycle of stimulation and pause multiple times, eventually increasing the length of each edging session. Focus on prolonging arousal and slowing ejaculation with each repeat.

Step 4: Communication and Collaboration: Communicate freely with your partner about learning the edging method together. Share your opinions, boundaries, and comments to ensure a mutually enjoyable experience.

Additional ideas for the Edging Technique:
Practice Edging: Edging includes bringing yourself to the brink of orgasm repeatedly before ejaculation. Start by stimulating yourself or your partner until you're close to climax, then pause or lower stimulation to avoid ejaculation. Repeat this cycle

multiple times to prolong arousal and improve sexual energy.

Communication is Key: Communicate with your partner about learning cutting together. Share your preferences and limits, and provide feedback to help each other measure arousal levels and change stimulation properly. This collaborative method can improve trust and intimacy while learning the edging technique.

7. Kegel Exercises:

Step 1: Identify Pelvic Floor Muscles: Begin by finding your pelvic floor muscles, which are the muscles you use to stop the flow of pee. Practice tightening and relaxing these muscles to familiarize yourself with their location and feeling.

Step 2: Perform Kegel Exercises: Once you've found your pelvic floor muscles, practice kegel exercises by tightening them for a few seconds, then relaxing for an equal length. Aim for several sets of repetitions each day to build power and stamina.

Step 3: Incorporate During Intimacy: During sexual action, engage your pelvic floor muscles to delay ejaculation. Experiment with different levels of muscle stress to find what works best for you and improves arousal without triggering ejaculation.

Step 4: Regular Practice and Communication: Make kegel exercises a regular part of your schedule and speak with your partner about your progress. Share your stories and work on ways to add pelvic floor exercises into your intimate times.

Additional insights for Kegel Exercises:
Strengthen Pelvic Floor Muscles: Kegel movements involve tightening and relaxing the pelvic floor muscles to improve control over ejaculation. Practice squeezing the muscles you would use to stop the flow of pee, keeping for a few seconds, and then releasing. Aim for several sets of repetitions each day to build strength and stamina in these muscles.

Incorporate During Intimacy: During sexual action, engage your pelvic floor muscles to prevent ejaculation. Experiment with different amounts of muscle stress to find what works best for you. Regular practice of kegel exercises can lead to better ejaculatory control and increased sexual happiness for both you and your partner.

8. Delay Sprays or Creams:

Step 1: Choose a Delay Product: Select a delay spray or cream that includes chemicals like lidocaine or benzocaine, which briefly desensitize the penis to delay ejaculation. Follow the manufacturer's guidelines carefully and choose a product that suits your wants and tastes.

Step 2: Apply Before Sexual Activity: Apply the delay spray or cream to the penis soon before sexual activity, following the suggested dosage and application directions given on the packaging.

Step 3: Allow Time to soak: Allow the product to soak into the skin for the stated amount of time before participating in sexual action. This ensures maximum efficiency and minimizes the risk of transferring the product to your partner.

Step 4: Communication and permission: Communicate with your partner about using delay sprays or creams and gain their permission before applying them. Be open about any possible side effects or sensations and change usage based on your partner's comfort level and preferences.

Additional thoughts for Delay Sprays or Creams: Explore Over-the-Counter Options: Consider using delay sprays or creams that contain chemicals like lidocaine or benzocaine to briefly desensitize the penis and delay ejaculation. Follow the manufacturer's instructions carefully and apply the product to the penis shortly before sexual action for best results.

Communicate with Your Partner: Discuss the use of delay sprays or creams with your partner beforehand to ensure shared knowledge and agreement. Be open about any possible side effects or sensations, and change usage based on your preferences and comfort levels.

By following these step-by-step steps for each successful delay tactic, you can enhance your ability to prolong arousal and delay ejaculation, leading to more satisfying sexual experiences for you and your partner. Experiment with different techniques and methods to find what works best for your unique tastes and needs, and don't fear speaking freely with your partner throughout the process.

## Chapter Eight:

## Lifestyle Changes

In the goal of ejaculation mastery and general sexual health, lifestyle plays a key part. Just as a well-tuned engine powers a smooth ride, lifestyle factors such as food, exercise, and sleep serve as the basis for optimal ejaculatory control and sexual energy. Understanding how these living choices affect your body and making positive changes can lead to improved sexual performance, happiness, and general well-being. In this overview, we will delve into the intricate interplay between lifestyle and ejaculatory control, giving tips to empower people to make educated choices that support their sexual health path.

### 1. Lifestyle Factors Impacting Ejaculatory Control

Imagine your body as a highly tuned instrument, with various lifestyle factors acting as the keys that can either balance or break ejaculatory control. Let's review three key aspects of lifestyle – diet, exercise, and sleep – and how they influence your ability to control ejaculation.

1. Diet:
Just like fuel for a car, the food you eat gives energy and nutrients that power your body's processes,

including sexual performance. A diet rich in whole foods such as fruits, veggies, lean proteins, and whole grains offers important nutrients like vitamins, minerals, and antioxidants that support general sexual health. On the other hand, eating excessive amounts of processed foods, sugars, and unhealthy fats can lead to inflammation, hormonal changes, and reduced sexual function. By nourishing your body with a healthy and nutritious diet, you provide the necessary building blocks for good ejaculatory control.

Let's explore how your food impacts your ability to keep control and enjoy satisfying sexual experiences.

1. Nourishing Nutrients:
Think of nutrient-rich foods like superheroes coming in to save the day. Foods rich in vitamins, minerals, and antioxidants act as the building blocks for a healthy body, including your reproductive system. Incorporating plenty of fruits, veggies, whole grains, lean proteins, and healthy fats into your diet provides important nutrients that support hormonal balance and nerve function, both of which are crucial for ejaculatory control.

2. Inflammation and Hormonal Balance: Picture inflammation as a villain causing damage on your body's processes. Diets high in processed foods, sugars, and unhealthy fats can promote inflammation, which affects hormonal balance and nerve signals involved in ejaculation. By choosing whole, unprocessed foods instead, you can reduce

inflammation and support a better hormonal balance, eventually improving ejaculatory control.

3. Hydration: Imagine hydration as the oil that keeps your engine running smoothly. Staying properly hydrated ensures optimal blood flow and nerve function, both of which are important for sexual performance and ejaculatory control. Aim to drink plenty of water throughout the day to keep hydration levels and support general sexual health.

4. Mindful Eating: Consider mindful eating as the secret ingredient that improves your meal experience. Paying attention to hunger cues, chewing slowly, and enjoying each bite can help avoid overeating and promote better digestion and nutrition intake. By tuning into your body's signs and enjoying your meals mindfully, you can make better food choices that support cjaculatory control.

5. Balance and Moderation: Think of balance and moderation as the keys to a well-oiled machine. While it's important to favor nutrient-dense foods, giving yourself the odd treat or indulgence can also be part of a balanced diet. The key is moderation – loving less healthy foods in moderation while mainly filling your body with wholesome, nourishing choices.

By viewing your diet as fuel for optimal sexual performance, you can make informed decisions that support ejaculatory control and general sexual health. Just as a high-quality fuel keeps your car going easily, a balanced diet fuels your body's performance in the bedroom, ensuring a satisfying and pleasurable experience for you and your partner.

2. Exercise:

Think of exercise as the engine that drives your sexual success. Regular physical exercise not only improves cardiovascular health and circulation but also boosts testosterone levels, enhances happiness, and reduces stress – all of which contribute to better ejaculatory control. Engaging in exercises such as cardio, strength training, and pelvic floor movements improves the muscles involved in ejaculation and promotes total sexual energy. Additionally, exercise releases endorphins, the body's natural feel-good hormones, which can relieve worry and stress that may lead to premature ejaculation.

Let's explore how exercise impacts your ability to keep control and improve sexual satisfaction.

1. Pelvic Floor Power: Visualize your pelvic floor muscles as the supporting cast of actors in the show of ejaculation. These muscles play a crucial part in managing the flow of urine, supporting pelvic organs, and controlling ejaculation. By adding pelvic floor movements, such as kegels, into your routine, you can strengthen these muscles and improve your ability to control ejaculation.

2. Core Strength and Stability: Think of your core muscles as the basis of your body's success. A strong and stable core not only improves posture and

balance but also increases pelvic stability during sexual action. Exercises that target the core, such as planks, bridges, and abdominal crunches, can indirectly support ejaculatory control by boosting pelvic stability and muscle endurance.

3. Cardiovascular Health: Picture your cardiovascular system as the engine that drives your body's function. Regular physical exercise, such as running, swimming, or riding, improves blood flow and circulation throughout your body, including to the groin area. Enhanced blood flow to the pelvic area supports erectile function and arousal, leading to better ejaculatory control and sexual satisfaction.

4. Flexibility and Range of Motion: Imagine flexibility as the fluidity that improves your body's actions. Stretching exercises, such as yoga or Pilates, improve flexibility and range of motion, allowing for greater comfort and agility during sexual action. By improving flexibility in the hips, pelvis, and lower back, you can explore a wider range of sexual positions and movements while keeping control over ejaculation.

5. Mind-Body link: Consider the mind-body link as the director directing your body's show. Mindfulness practices, such as tai chi or meditation, foster awareness and presence in the moment, allowing you to tune into feelings and control arousal levels during sexual activity. By harnessing the power of your mind, you can improve ejaculatory control and increase pleasure.

By incorporating exercise into your lifestyle, you can strengthen your pelvic floor muscles, improve cardiovascular health, enhance flexibility, and develop a stronger mind-body link – all of which contribute to better ejaculatory control and sexual satisfaction. Just as regular practice refines singing skills, constant exercise hones your body's ability to perform best in the bedroom, ensuring a harmonious and happy sexual experience for you and your partner.

3. Sleep:
Consider sleep as the reset button for your body and mind. Quality sleep is important for hormonal balance, energy repair, and general well-being, all of which play a crucial part in ejaculatory control. Lack of sleep or poor sleep quality can disrupt hormonal balance, increase stress levels, and impair brain function, all of which can negatively impact sexual performance. Aim for 7-9 hours of restful sleep per night to help your body to recover and improve its processes, including sexual health.

Let's delve into how sleep impacts your ability to control arousal and improve sexual pleasure.

1. Restorative Repose: Visualize sleep as the time when your body undergoes repair and rebirth, like a magical potion that returns energy and strength. During sleep, your body fixes tissues, balances hormones, and restores energy stores, all of which are important for sexual health and function.

Adequate rest ensures that your body is prepped and ready for ideal sexual function.

2. Hormonal Harmony: Think of sleep as the director arranging your body's hormonal symphony. Adequate sleep controls hormone production, including testosterone, which plays a key role in sexual drive and function. Disrupted sleep habits can upset hormonal balance, leading to reduced libido and erectile failure, affecting ejaculatory control.

3. Stress Reduction: Picture sleep as the antidote to stress, a relaxing balm that calms the nervous system and returns mental balance. Quality sleep lowers cortisol levels, the stress hormone, and promotes relaxation, which is important for good sexual performance. High stress levels can lead to worry, performance pressure, and premature ejaculation, showing the importance of restful sleep in managing ejaculatory control.

4. Mental Clarity and Focus: Consider sleep as the reset button for your brain, allowing you to wake up refreshed, alert, and mentally sharp. Adequate sleep improves brain function, memory storage, and decision-making skills, all of which are vital for keeping focus and control during sexual activity. Fatigue and sleep deprivation can impair brain performance and reduce ejaculatory control.

5. Emotional Well-being: Imagine sleep as the refuge where emotional resilience is developed and reinforced. Quality sleep improves mood, lowers irritability, and supports mental stability, encouraging a positive attitude and healthy interpersonal relationships. Emotional well-being is closely linked to sexual pleasure and ejaculatory control, stressing the importance of restorative sleep for general sexual health.

By valuing quality sleep and adopting healthy sleep habits, such as keeping a regular sleep schedule, creating a relaxing bedtime routine, and improving your sleep surroundings, you can improve ejaculatory control and enhance sexual energy. Just as a well-tuned instrument makes beautiful music, a well-rested body and mind work harmoniously in the bedroom, ensuring a fulfilling and satisfying sexual experience for you and your partner.

By paying attention to these lifestyle factors – nourishing your body with healthy foods, staying physically active, and valuing quality sleep – you can empower yourself to take control of your ejaculatory function and improve your overall sexual experience. Just as a well-tuned instrument makes beautiful music, a balanced lifestyle promotes optimal ejaculatory control and sexual pleasure.

## 2. Revitalize Your Sexual Health: Lifestyle Tips for Enhanced Stamina

Embarking on a journey to bolster your sexual health and energy is akin to growing a blooming plant – it requires nurturing care, commitment, and a sprinkle of creativity. Let's explore some suggestions for making positive lifestyle changes to elevate your sexual well-being and stamina, given in simple terms for easy implementation:

1. Nutrition Nourishment:
Imagine your body as a beautiful castle, reinforced by the nutrients you provide it. Just like a castle needs sturdy walls and a well-stocked kitchen to grow, your body relies on nourishing foods to fuel its energy and strength. Let's dive into the world of nutrition nourishment, where we'll explore simple yet powerful ways to boost your sexual health and stamina:

1. Powerful Proteins: Think of proteins as the heroes in shining armor, protecting your body against tiredness and weakness. Incorporate lean forms of protein such as chicken, fish, eggs, and beans into your meals to support muscle power and endurance. These mighty fighters will fortify your body for the tasks ahead, ensuring you have the energy to conquer any quest.

2. Mighty Minerals and Vitamins: Imagine minerals and vitamins as the magical potions that give energy and strength upon your kingdom. Fill your plate with a

colorful array of fruits and veggies, rich in important vitamins and minerals like vitamin C, vitamin E, zinc, and selenium. These enchanted elixirs will strengthen your immune system, improve blood flow, and fuel your body with the energy needed for epic adventures between the sheets.

3. Hydration Heroes: Picture water as the life-giving elixir that quenches your body's thirst and supports its vigor. Just as a well runs with refreshing water to feed the land, your body grows when hydrated. Sip on water throughout the day like a noble knight quenching his thirst at a crystal-clear stream, keeping your body hydrated and ready for action.

4. Wise Whole Grains: Envision whole grains as the hearty bread that supports your health and resilience. Swap sweetened carbs for whole grains like quinoa, brown rice, and oats to provide your body with a steady source of energy. These wholesome grains will feed your body like a roaring fire, keeping you warm and energized throughout your travels.

5. Fruitful Fats: Imagine healthy fats as the secret wealth hidden within the kingdom, ready to be found and enjoyed. Incorporate sources of healthy fats such as eggs, nuts, seeds, and olive oil into your diet to feed your body and support natural balance. These precious fats will provide steady energy and improve your body's resilience, ensuring you're ready to face whatever challenges come your way.

Incorporating these nutrition nourishment tactics into your daily life is like strengthening the walls of your castle, ensuring that your body stays strong, adaptable, and ready for adventure. With the power of nutritious foods by your side, you'll start on a trip of energy and strength, ruling the realm of sexual health with confidence and vigor.

2. Exercise Excellence:

Picture your body as a beautiful country, bustling with activity and energy. Just as a kingdom thrives with movement and energy, your body flourishes with exercise greatness. Let's start on a journey through the world of fitness, where we'll discover simple yet powerful ways to improve your sexual health and stamina:

1. Mighty Muscles: Envision your muscles as the loyal heroes of your country, strong and resilient in the face of obstacles. Engage in strength-training exercises such as lifting weights, bodyweight exercises, or resistance band workouts to build your muscles and improve endurance. These noble heroes will fortify your body, improving your ability to perform with energy and stamina.

2. Cardiovascular Crusades: Imagine cardiovascular workouts as the great quests that invigorate your body and spirit. Engage in sports like jogging, swimming, riding, or dancing to raise your heart rate and improve circulation. These exhilarating adventures will enhance your cardiovascular health,

better blood flow to all parts of your body, including those important for sexual performance.

3. Flexibility and Fluidity: Picture flexibility exercises as the graceful moves that promote quickness and suppleness. Incorporate activities like yoga, Pilates, or stretching routines to improve flexibility and movement. These fluid movements will improve your range of motion and reduce the risk of harm, allowing you to move with ease and grace during intimate meetings.

4. Endurance Expeditions: Envision endurance workouts as epic trips that test your strength and stamina. Engage in sports like hiking, running, or riding to build strength and resilience. These endurance adventures will test your body and mind, preparing you for the long haul and ensuring you have the endurance to enjoy prolonged closeness.

5. Mind-Body Mastery: Imagine mind-body movements as the ancient skills that join body and spirit in unity. Practice activities like tai chi, qigong, or thoughtful meditation to develop inner calm and balance. These mindful routines will sharpen your focus, reduce stress, and enhance your general well-being, allowing you to approach intimacy with a clear and centered mind.

By adding these exercise excellence techniques into your daily routine, you'll release the full potential of your body and mind, starting on a quest for sexual health and stamina with courage and drive. With each step and each rep, you'll strengthen your body, invigorate your spirit, and open the key to permanent energy and vigor in the realm of intimacy.

3. Sleep Sanctuary:
Imagine your bedroom as a sanctuary, a calm place where you escape each night to rest and refresh. Just as a refuge provides comfort for the weary soul, prioritizing quality sleep turns your bedroom into a Sleep refuge, nurturing your body and mind for optimal sexual health and energy. Let's explore how to develop this holy space:

1. Pillows of Peace: Picture your pillows as fluffy clouds, supporting your head and neck in heavenly ease. Invest in supportive pillows that align your spine and promote proper alignment, ensuring you wake up refreshed and free from pain or soreness. These pillows of peace will surround you in calm, inviting restorative sleep.

2. Cozy Comforters: Envision your blanket as a soft cocoon, covering you in warmth and protection as you drift into dreamland. Choose beds made from breathable, natural fabrics like cotton or bamboo to control temperature and promote restful sleep. With each gentle hug, your cozy blanket lulls you into a state of deep relaxation, preparing you for restorative rest.

3. Soothing melody: Imagine a tranquil melody filling your Sleep Sanctuary, immersing you in a song of peace. Explore relaxing sounds such as nature sounds, white noise, or calming music to drown out distractions and promote restful sleep. These melodic tunes will take you to a state of tranquility, easing your mind and lulling you into peaceful sleep.

4. Dimmed Lighting: Picture soft, dimmed lighting creating a nice glow throughout your Sleep Sanctuary, signaling to your body that it's time to relax and prepare for sleep. Opt for changeable lighting options such as bedside lamps or dimmer switches to create a cozy environment beneficial to rest. As the lights slowly fade, your body and mind surrender to the soothing embrace of darkness, bringing in restful sleep.

5. Digital Detox: Envision your Sleep Sanctuary as a technology-free zone, free from the distractions of computers and gadgets that disturb your sleep-wake cycle. Establish a bedtime practice that includes unplugging from electronic devices at least an hour before sleep, allowing your mind to unwind and prepare for rest. With each digital detox, you reclaim your Sleep Sanctuary as a holy place for rejuvenation and rebirth.

By transforming your bedroom into a Sleep Sanctuary, you create an environment that supports deep, restorative sleep, replenishing your energy stores and improving your sexual health and vigor. With each night spent in this tranquil haven, you awaken feeling refreshed, revived, and ready to embrace the day with increased energy and vitality.


4. Stress Management Strategies:
Imagine worry as a twisted knot, wrapping around you like a constricting snake, draining your energy and clouding your mind. But fear not, for within the labyrinth of stress lies a road to serenity, illuminated by stress management techniques that enable you to retake control and restore balance to your life. Let's unravel this knot together, discovering creative and simple ways to handle stress:

1. Mindful Breathing: Close your eyes and picture yourself standing on the side of a calm lake, the gentle rhythm of your breath matching the ebb and flow of the water. Take slow, deep breaths, inhaling peace and exhaling stress with each focused breath. As you immerse yourself in the current moment, the waves of stress eventually subside, leaving behind a sense of peace and clarity.

2. Nature Retreat: Picture yourself walking through a lush forest, surrounded by towering trees and colorful leaves that dance in the breeze. Step outside and immerse yourself in nature's embrace, allowing the sights, sounds, and smells of the natural world to soothe your mind. Whether you stroll through a park, hike a wooded trail, or simply bask in the warmth of

the sun, nature offers a haven where stress melts away like morning dew.

3. Creative Expression: Envision yourself as an artist, holding a brush or pen to channel your feelings onto a blank wall or page. Engage in artistic activities such as drawing, writing, or crafting, allowing your deepest thoughts and feelings to take shape in tangible form. As you unleash your imagination, you release pent-up stress and find comfort in the act of self-expression.
4. Movement Meditation: Imagine yourself as a dancer, moving smoothly to the rhythm of your own heartbeat, releasing stress with each fluid motion. Engage in focused movement practices such as yoga, tai chi, or qigong, connecting mind, body, and spirit through slow, flowing movements. As you match breath with movement, you develop a sense of inner calm and balance that transcends the chaos of daily life.

5. Gratitude Practice: Close your eyes and imagine a radiant sun, sending its golden rays upon fields of blooming flowers, each petal aglow with gratitude. Cultivate a daily practice of thankfulness, reflecting on the blessings and wealth in your life, no matter how small. Whether you keep a gratitude book, offer silent thanks before meals, or simply pause to appreciate the beauty around you, gratitude illuminates the darkness of stress, creating a sense of peace and contentment.

By embracing these creative and easy stress management strategies, you empower yourself to handle life's obstacles with resilience and grace. With each mindful breath, nature retreat, artistic expression, movement meditation, and moment of thanks, you pave the way to a life filled with calm, joy, and inner peace.

5. Communication and Connection:

Imagine conversation and connection as the threads that knit the fabric of your relationships, linking you to others in a tapestry of understanding and support. Let's explore how you can improve these vital parts creatively and simply:

1. Heartfelt Conversations: Picture yourself sitting across from a loved one, the warmth of their presence covering you like a cozy blanket on a cold day. Engage in heartfelt conversations where you share your thoughts, feelings, and goals freely and honestly. Listen carefully to their words, giving understanding and validation, as you create deeper connections through the power of authentic communication.

2. Quality Time Together: Envision yourself going on a shared journey with your loved ones, whether it's a leisurely walk in the park, a cozy movie night at home, or an unexpected road trip to new places. Make time to nurture your relationships by prioritizing valuable time together, free from distractions and responsibilities. By creating important events and memories, you strengthen the bonds that unite you, fostering a sense of connection and belonging.

3. Expressing Appreciation: Imagine yourself as a light of gratitude, shining bright with appreciation for the people who improve your life. Take moments to show your thanks and appreciation for your loved ones, whether through heartfelt words, thoughtful gestures, or small acts of kindness. By recognizing the value they bring to your life, you affirm the strength of your relationship and create a culture of mutual respect and support.

4. Active Listening: See yourself as a compassionate listener, giving the gift of your presence and undivided attention to those who seek comfort in your company. Practice active listening by fully connecting with others when they speak, setting aside distractions and opinions to truly understand their perspective. Through active listening, you support their experiences and emotions, encouraging stronger relationships built on trust and understanding.

5. Shared Experiences: Envision yourself going on shared experiences and journeys with your loved ones, building memories that will last a lifetime. Whether it's exploring new hobbies together, going on outdoor trips, or simply enjoying meals as a family, shared experiences strengthen the bonds that unite you. By engaging in activities that bring joy and satisfaction to both parties, you strengthen your connection and build a foundation of shared experiences to value.

By adopting these creative and simple strategies for communication and connection, you improve your relationships and foster stronger bonds with the people who matter most in your life. Through heartfelt talks, valuable time together, expressions of praise, active listening, and shared experiences, you build a tapestry of connection that withstands the tests of time and strengthens with each passing moment.

By following these lifestyle tips with creativity and commitment, you can revitalize your sexual health and stamina, unlocking new levels of vitality and happiness in the bedroom. Just as a well-tended plant grows with care and attention, your sexual well-being will blossom with the nurturing support of positive lifestyle changes.

# Chapter Nine:

## Mental Rehearsal and Visualization

Welcome to the world of mental practice and visualization, where the power of your mind becomes the key to achieving greater control and mastery over your sexual experiences. In this enchanted space, we'll journey together through the realms of fantasy and inner discovery, finding the transformative potential of controlling your thoughts and beliefs. Through the old arts of mental practice and visualization, you'll learn to shape your reality, shaping your sexual experiences with meaning and purpose. Join us as we start on a quest to elevate your sexual performance and unlock new realms of pleasure and satisfaction.

### 1. Mental Rehearsal Techniques

Mental practice methods are like rehearsals before a big show, but instead of a stage, you're preparing your mind and body for the complex dance of sexual intimacy. Here's a clever and simple breakdown of how these methods work:

1. Visualization:
Visualization is a strong mental method that involves making vivid mental pictures or scenes to achieve a desired result. When it comes to improving ejaculatory control, visualization can be an effective

tool for teaching the mind to react calmly and proudly during sexual meetings. Here's a thorough breakdown of how visualization works and how to add it into your routine:

1. Setting the Scene:
- Find a quiet and comfortable place where you can relax without distractions.
- Close your eyes and take a few deep breaths to calm yourself and clear your mind.
- Begin to imagine yourself in a sexual scenario, either with your partner or in a solo situation.

2. Creating the Scenario:
- Imagine the scene in detail, including the location, lighting, and any other sensory elements that add to the experience.
- Visualize yourself and your partner, or the desired sexual situation, with as much clarity and reality as possible.
- Picture the feelings, movements, and emotions involved in the sexual encounter, focused on staying relaxed and in control throughout.

3. Maintaining Control:
- As you imagine the scene developing, pay attention to your level of arousal and any feelings of stress or worry that appear.
- If you notice feelings of arousal rising too quickly, imagine yourself taking conscious steps to maintain control. This could involve slowing down the pace,

focusing on your breath, or shifting your attention to other feelings or thoughts.
- Visualize yourself successfully controlling your arousal and lengthening the sexual experience, feeling confident and powerful in your ability to do so.

4. Repetition and Practice:
- Repeat this visualization exercise regularly, ideally as part of a daily practice or before engaging in sexual action.
- The more you practice meditation, the more effective it becomes at teaching your mind to react calmly and confidently during real sexual experiences.

- Over time, you'll find that the mental imagery you create during visualization matches more closely with your experiences in real life, improving your ability to control arousal and prolong pleasure.

5. Integration with Other Techniques:
- Visualization can be combined with other methods, such as deep breathing or progressive muscle relaxation, to increase its usefulness.
- For example, you can add visualization into a bigger relaxation practice, using mental images to guide your body into a state of calm and focus.

By adding visualization into your routine and performing it regularly, you can train your mind to respond more effectively to sexual stimulation and keep control over ejaculation.

2. Positive Affirmations:
Positive affirmations are strong statements that can help change negative beliefs and support positive attitudes and behaviors. When it comes to improving ejaculatory control, happy mantras can be a valuable tool for building confidence and self-assurance. Here's a full description of how positive affirmations work and how to add them into your routine:

1. Understanding Positive Affirmations:
- Positive affirmations are short, simple statements that support positive traits or results.
- They work by influencing your subconscious mind, gradually reshaping your views and behaviors over time.
- By saying positive affirmations regularly, you can improve your belief in your ability to achieve your goals.

2. Creating Effective Affirmations:
- When creating positive words for ejaculatory control, focus on statements that stress your ability to maintain control and lengthen pleasure.
- Keep statements concise, detailed, and in the present tense. For example, "I am in control of my pleasure" or "I can last as long as I want."
- Choose affirmations that connect with you personally and feel powerful when repeated.

3. Incorporating Affirmations into Your Routine:
- Set aside specific time each day to practice mantras, such as in the morning upon waking or before bed.

- Find a quiet and comfy place where you can focus without distractions.
- Close your eyes and say your chosen affirmations loudly or quietly to yourself.
- Visualize the statements as true and allow yourself to feel the feelings connected with them, such as confidence and strength.
- Repeat each affirmation multiple times, focused on the meaning and purpose behind the words.

4. Consistency and Repetition:
- Consistency is key when it comes to using mantras successfully. Aim to practice them daily, ideally multiple times a day.
- Repetition helps strengthen the messages found within the affirmations, gradually changing your thinking and beliefs.
- Over time, you'll begin to absorb the affirmations, leading to greater confidence and belief in your ability to achieve ejaculatory control.

5. Integration with Other Techniques:
- Affirmations can be combined with other techniques for better ejaculatory control, such as visualization or relaxation routines.
- Incorporate mantras into your relaxing routine or vision practice to improve their usefulness.
- By combining affirmations with other methods, you can create a complete approach to building confidence and control over ejaculation.

By incorporating positive mantras into your daily routine and repeating them repeatedly, you can develop an attitude of confidence and strength, increasing your ability to achieve ejaculatory control and prolong pleasure.

3. Mindfulness Practice:
Mindfulness practice involves staying fully present in the moment, aware of your feelings, thoughts, and emotions without judgment. When it comes to improving ejaculatory control, mindfulness can be a valuable tool for reducing worry and distraction, allowing you to keep focus and manage arousal more effectively.
Here's a thorough description of how to add mindfulness into your routine:

1. Understanding Mindfulness:
- Mindfulness is the practice of deliberately paying attention to the current moment, with an attitude of openness, curiosity, and acceptance.
- It includes watching your thoughts, feelings, and bodily sensations without getting caught up in them or responding automatically.
- By developing mindfulness, you can develop greater self-awareness and the ability to react carefully to difficult situations, including sexual meetings.

2. Practicing Mindfulness During Sexual Activity:
- Start by setting aside any expectations or judgments about your behavior or the result of the sexual experience.

- Focus on the physical feelings in your body, such as the touch of your partner's skin, the beat of your breath, and the movement of your muscles.
- Notice any thoughts or feelings that come without getting carried away by them. If distracting thoughts appear, gently bring your attention back to the present moment.
- Stay connected with your partner by keeping eye contact, speaking freely, and tuning into their reactions and needs.
- Allow yourself to fully feel the pleasure and intimacy of the moment without thinking about reaching a specific goal or result.

3. Cultivating Mindfulness Outside of Sexual Activity:
- Practice mindfulness meditation daily to improve your ability to stay present and focused.
- Set aside committed time each day for regular meditation practice, starting with just a few minutes and gradually increasing the length over time.
- Incorporate casual awareness techniques into your daily routine, such as thoughtful eating, walking, or breathing exercises.
- Use awareness methods to handle stress and anxiety in other areas of your life, as lowering general stress can also positively impact sexual function and performance.

4. Integration with Other Techniques:
- Mindfulness can be combined with other techniques for better ejaculatory control, such as visualization, relaxation exercises, and positive affirmations.

- Combine awareness with deep breathing or
progressive muscle relaxation methods to improve
relaxation and reduce stress in the body.
- Use mindfulness to help reframe any negative
thoughts or beliefs about sexual performance,
creating a more positive and accepting attitude
towards yourself and your skills.

By practicing mindfulness during sexual activity and
adding it into your daily routine, you can develop
greater self-awareness, reduce worry and distraction,
and improve your ability to control arousal and
lengthen pleasure.

4. Progressive Muscle Relaxation:
Progressive muscle relaxation is a method that
involves gradually tensing and then relaxing different
muscle groups in your body to release stress and
promote relaxation. Here's a thorough description of
how to practice progressive muscle relaxation to
improve ejaculatory control:

1. Understanding Progressive Muscle Relaxation:
- Progressive muscle relaxation (PMR) is a relaxation
method created by American physician Edmund
Jacobson in the early 20th century.
- The method involves tensing specific muscle groups
in your body for a few seconds, then releasing the
tension and allowing the muscles to rest fully.
- By carefully tensing and relaxing each muscle group,
you can increase awareness of stress in your body
and learn to release it more effectively.

2. Practicing Progressive Muscle Relaxation:
- Find a quiet and comfortable place where you can lie down or sit in a relaxed position.
- Close your eyes and take a few deep breaths to calm yourself and prepare for the practice.
- Begin by focusing on your toes. Curl them tightly and hold the tightness for a few seconds, then release and allow them to relax fully.
- Move on to the muscles in your feet and legs, tensing them quickly before releasing and relaxing.
- Continue this process, working your way up through your legs, thighs, buttocks, belly, chest, arms, hands, neck, and face, tensing and releasing each muscle group in turn.
- As you tense each muscle group, focus on the feeling of tension rising and then melting away as you release the tension.
- Take your time with each muscle group, allowing yourself to fully feel the relaxation reaction before going on to the next.

3. Benefits for Ejaculatory Control:
- Progressive muscle relaxation can help reduce general stress and tension in your body, making it easier to stay cool and collected during sexual activity.

- By practicing PMR regularly, you can increase your awareness of stress in your body and learn to release it more effectively, which can help you stay relaxed and in control during intimate times.

- Relaxing your muscles can also promote better blood flow to the groin area, which may enhance sexual desire and improve ejaculatory control.

4. Integration with Other Techniques:
- Progressive muscle relaxation can be combined with other relaxation methods, such as deep breathing or visualization, to increase its usefulness.
- Incorporate PMR into your daily routine, either as a solo exercise or as part of a bigger relaxation session.

- Use PMR before sexual action to help calm your nerves and reduce performance anxiety, allowing you to focus more fully on the feelings and pleasure of the experience.

By practicing progressive muscle relaxation regularly, you can reduce overall stress in your body, promote relaxation, and improve your ability to stay calm and composed during sexual activity, eventually improving your ejaculatory control and overall sexual pleasure.

5. Guided Imagery:
Guided imagery is a strong method that involves listening to tapes or scripts meant to lead you through visualizations aimed at promoting relaxation and confidence. Here's a detailed description of how guided imagery can help improve ejaculatory control:

1. Understanding Guided Imagery:
- Guided imagery is a relaxation method that uses the power of visualization to create a feeling of calm and focus.
- During guided imagery classes, you listen to tapes or texts that guide you through a number of mental pictures and situations meant to evoke feelings of relaxation and confidence.
- These guided experiences often combine soothing imagery, calming music, and positive affirmations to help you reach a state of deep relaxation and mental focus.

2. Practicing Guided Imagery:
- Find a quiet and comfortable place where you won't be disturbed, and choose a guided imagery recording or script that works with you.
- Close your eyes and take a few deep breaths to calm yourself and prepare for the visualization practice.
- Listen to the recording or read the script, allowing yourself to fully immerse in the images and feelings described.
- Visualize yourself in a calm and quiet setting, such as a beach, forest, or hill, and imagine feeling completely relaxed and at ease.
- Focus on the details of the scene, including sounds, smells, and feelings, allowing yourself to become fully absorbed in the experience.
- As you listen to the guided imagery, pay attention to any feelings of stress or worry melting away, replaced by a sense of calm and confidence.
3. Benefits for Ejaculatory Control:

- Guided imagery can be a strong tool for boosting relaxation and reducing stress, both of which are key factors in ejaculatory control.
- By regularly performing guided imagery, you can train your mind to respond more effectively to sexual stimulation and keep control over ejaculation.
- The relaxing images and positive mantras used in guided imagery sessions can help improve your confidence and self-esteem, allowing you to approach sexual activity with a greater sense of ease and security.

4. Integration with Other Techniques:
- Guided imagery can be used on its own or in combination with other relaxing methods, such as deep breathing or progressive muscle relaxation, to improve its usefulness.
- Incorporate guided images into your daily routine, listening to tapes or reading lines regularly to promote relaxation and mental focus.
- Use guided images before sexual activity to help calm your jitters and reduce performance anxiety, allowing you to approach intimate times with greater confidence and control.

By incorporating guided imagery into your routine and practicing regularly, you can promote relaxation, boost confidence, and improve your ability to keep control over ejaculation during sexual activity, eventually improving your general sexual satisfaction and well-being.

By adding these mental rehearsal methods into your routine, you can train your mind to work in harmony with your body, improving your ability to control arousal and increase sexual pleasure.

## 2. Visualization Exercises to Reframe Thoughts and Beliefs About Sexual Performance

Visualization exercises are strong tools that can help change thoughts and beliefs about sexual performance, boosting confidence, and improving ejaculatory control. Here's a complete guide to imagination exercises:

1. Understanding Visualization:
Visualization is like making a movie in your head. It's when you picture things in your head to help you imagine getting something you want.

When you do visualization exercises, you imagine yourself doing things the way you want them to go. For example, in the setting of sex, you might imagine yourself staying calm and in control during closeness.

2. Setting the Stage:
- Find a quiet, comfy spot where you won't be bothered.
- Close your eyes and take a few deep breaths to relax.
- Picture a calm place in your mind, like a peaceful beach or a quiet forest. This helps you feel relaxed and focused for meditation practice.

3. Creating the Scene:
- Imagine yourself in a sexual setting where you usually feel anxious or fight to keep control.
- Picture the surroundings, your partner's presence, and the feelings you generally feel during intimacy.
- Make the visualization complete, including sights, sounds, smells, and feelings, to make it feel real and vivid.

4. Positive Reinforcement:
- Imagine yourself easily navigating the scene, keeping control over your arousal.
- Visualize staying relaxed, focused, and loving the experience without feeling stressed.
- Use positive affirmations or self-talk to improve your confidence and support your belief in your ability to control ejaculation.

5. Repetition and Practice:
- Make visualization a regular practice to strengthen good views about sexual success.
- Before engaging in sexual action, use visualization to calm jitters and reduce performance anxiety.
- Employ visualization as a mental practice method to prepare for difficult scenarios and reinforce desired behaviors and outcomes.

6. Integration with Other Techniques:
- Combine visualization with relaxation methods like deep breathing or progressive muscle relaxation to improve its usefulness.

- Make visualization a part of your daily routine,
spending a few minutes each day picturing great
results and keeping control over ejaculation.
- Use visualization to challenge and replace negative
ideas or beliefs about sexual performance with
positive, empowering pictures and statements.

By adding visualization exercises into your routine and
practicing regularly, you can reframe negative
thoughts and beliefs about sexual performance,
promote confidence, and improve ejaculatory control,
eventually leading to a more enjoyable and fulfilling
sexual experience.

# Chapter Ten:

## Overcoming Challenges

In our journey towards learning ejaculation control, we face various challenges and failures along the way. These hurdles can sometimes feel overwhelming, but they are all part of the process of growth and learning. In this part, we'll explore how to face these challenges head-on, with strategies to stay inspired and determined. By knowing and addressing these obstacles, we can pave the way for long-term success in meeting our goals of ejaculation mastery. So, let's dive in and discover how to beat these hurdles together!

## 1. Common Obstacles and Setbacks in Mastering Ejaculation Control

Addressing common hurdles and failures in learning ejaculation control is like navigating through rough seas on a boat. Along the trip, we may face different challenges that test our resolve and drive. One common challenge is performance anxiety, where worrying about pleasing our partner or meeting unrealistic standards can lead to premature ejaculation. Another setback is lack of communication, as addressing sensitive subjects like sexual performance may feel uncomfortable. Additionally, distractions, such as stress from work or daily life, can break our attention during intimate times.

To conquer these obstacles, it's important to create a supportive and understanding environment with our partner. Open conversation is key to handling worries and fears, allowing us to work together as a team. Building trust and closeness in the relationship creates a safe place where we can freely talk about challenges and explore answers together.

Practicing relaxation methods, such as deep breathing or awareness, helps calm our nerves and reduce nervousness during sexual action. By staying present in the moment and focusing on feelings rather than worries, we can lengthen the experience and delay ejaculation.

Moreover, incorporating lifestyle changes like regular exercise, healthy eating habits, and proper sleep can improve general sexual health and stamina. These lifestyle changes add to our physical and mental well-being, enhancing our ability to control ejaculation.

It's important to remember that beating barriers takes time and patience. Celebrate small wins along the way and stay inspired by setting realistic goals. With persistence and a positive attitude, we can beat obstacles and achieve mastery over ejaculation control, leading to a more fulfilling and satisfying sex life.

Common hurdles and setbacks in learning ejaculation control include:

1. Performance anxiety: Worrying about pleasing your partner or meeting high standards can lead to premature ejaculation.

Remedy:
Practice relaxation methods such as deep breathing or awareness to calm nerves and reduce nervousness during sexual activity. Open conversation with your partner about fears and worries can also alleviate performance pressure.

2. Lack of communication: Avoiding discussions about sexual performance or problems may hinder progress in handling ejaculation control issues.

Remedy:
Foster open and honest conversation with your partner about sensitive topics related to sexual health. Create a welcoming atmosphere where both partners feel comfortable sharing their wants and concerns.

3. Distractions: Stress from work, daily life, or intrusive thoughts during private moments can break focus and add to premature ejaculation.

Remedy:
Practice mindfulness methods to stay present in the moment and shift attention away from distractions.

Engage in activities that encourage relaxation and stress release, such as exercise or sports, to improve general mental well-being.

4. Physical factors: Underlying medical problems, chemical changes, or medicines may affect ejaculatory control.

Remedy:
Consult with a healthcare worker to rule out any medical issues adding to ejaculation problems. Explore treatment choices or lifestyle changes that can address root causes and improve sexual health.

5. Lack of information or skills: Limited understanding of ejaculation control methods or lack of practice may impede progress in mastering control.

Remedy:
Educate yourself about useful techniques for slowing ejaculation, such as the stop-start method or squeeze technique. Practice these methods daily and seek help from a therapist or sex trainer if needed.

6. Unrealistic expectations: Believing that you should be able to last forever or comparing yourself to unrealistic standards presented in the media can cause pressure and anger.

Remedy:
Set realistic standards for yourself and your sexual encounters. Remember that every individual's body

and reaction to input are unique. Focus on progress rather than perfection, enjoying small wins along the way.

7. Lack of self-awareness: Not being sensitive to your body's cues or knowing your arousal patterns can make it challenging to control ejaculation.

Remedy:
Practice self-awareness methods such as mindfulness or writing to track arousal levels and find causes for premature ejaculation. Pay attention to subtle changes in feeling and learn to recognize when you're reaching the point of no return.

8. Inconsistent practice: Irregular or occasional practice of ejaculation control methods may limit progress and effectiveness.

Remedy:
Establish a constant practice routine for adopting ejaculation control techniques, such as booking regular practice sessions or combining techniques into your sexual meetings with your partner. Consistency is key to building and keeping ejaculatory control over time.

9. Relationship issues: Relationship problems, unresolved tensions, or lack of emotional link with your partner can impact sexual function and ejaculation control.

Remedy:
Prioritize nurturing your relationship and handling any underlying problems or tensions that may be hurting closeness. Invest time and effort in building trust, communication, and emotional link with your partner, as a helpful and harmonious relationship can contribute to better sexual happiness and control.

10. Impatience or frustration: Feeling frustrated or impatient with slow progress in learning ejaculation control can lead to feelings of frustration or inadequacy.

Remedy:
Practice self-compassion and patience throughout your road to learning ejaculation control. Recognize that change takes time and effort, and failures are a normal part of the process. Celebrate your successes and milestones along the way, no matter how small, and keep a positive view on your progress.

11. Negative self-talk: Engaging in negative self-talk or holding beliefs of inadequacy can weaken confidence and self-esteem, impacting your ability to control ejaculation.

Remedy:
Challenge and change negative thoughts or beliefs about your sexual skills and abilities. Practice self-affirmations and positive self-talk to develop an attitude of confidence and self-assurance. Focus on your strengths and successes rather than dwelling on

perceived flaws or mistakes, creating a more positive and empowering attitude on your journey towards mastering ejaculation control.

12. Lack of support: Trying to improve ejaculation control without the help of your partner or a supportive social network can make the process more difficult.

Remedy:
Seek help from your partner, friends, or support groups who can offer motivation, understanding, and useful advice. Share your goals and success with your partner, and involve them in your journey towards learning ejaculation control. A helpful and collaborative approach can improve your bond with your partner and provide priceless support as you handle challenges and setbacks along the way.

By handling these common hurdles and failures with appropriate remedies, people can enhance their ability to master ejaculation control and enjoy more satisfying sexual experiences.

## 2. Strategies for Staying Motivated and Persistent in Achieving Long-term Success.

Staying inspired and persistent in achieving long-term success in learning ejaculation control is crucial for beating obstacles and reaching your goals. Here are some creative yet easy methods to help you stay on track:

1. Set Clear Goals:
Define specific, measured, and realistic goals related
to ejaculation control, such as staying a certain length
during intercourse or learning specific methods. Break
down large goals into smaller steps to track progress
and celebrate wins along the way.
Setting clear goals is important for learning
ejaculation control.

Here's how to grow and explore this strategy:

1. Define Specific Goals: Start by finding what you
want to achieve in terms of ejaculation control. This
could include lasting longer during intercourse,
lowering performance anxiety, or learning specific
techniques like the stop-start method or the squeeze
technique.

2. Make Goals Measurable: Ensure that your goals are
measured so that you can track your growth over
time. For example, you might aim to increase your
length of intercourse from a few minutes to a certain
number of minutes or to hit a specific level of arousal
before ejaculating.

3. Ensure Goals are Achievable: Set realistic goals
that you think you can achieve with effort and
dedication. Avoid making goals that are too ambitious
or unrealistic, as this can lead to anger and
disappointment.

4. Break Down Goals into Milestones: Divide bigger goals into smaller, more doable milestones. For example, if your final goal is to last 15 minutes during intercourse, you might set targets to last 5 minutes, then 7 minutes, then 10 minutes, and so on. This makes the process feel more achievable and helps you to enjoy progress along the way.

5. Track Progress: Keep track of your progress towards your goals by recording your performance during sexual encounters or practice sessions. Use a journal or a tracking app to record your length of intercourse, arousal levels, and any methods or strategies you're using.

6. Celebrate Achievements: Celebrate each milestone you hit along the way to achieving your bigger goals. Recognize and thank yourself for your progress, whether it's with a small treat, a night out, or simply recognizing your successes.

7. Adjust Goals as Needed: Be open and ready to adjust your goals based on your experiences and progress. If you find that a particular goal is too challenging or not challenging enough, don't hesitate to change it properly. The key is to keep going forward and staying motivated towards your final goal of mastering ejaculation control.

2. Visualize Success:
Use the power of visualization to imagine yourself achieving your goals and feeling the benefits of better ejaculation control. Create vivid mental pictures of great results, focusing on the feelings of satisfaction, confidence, and intimacy that follow control.

Visualizing success is a strong method for staying motivated and persistent in achieving long-term success in mastering ejaculation control.

Here's how to grow and explore this strategy:

1. Create Vivid Mental Images: Take time each day to picture yourself achieving your goals linked to ejaculation control. Close your eyes and imagine a situation where you successfully last longer during intercourse or effectively use techniques to delay ejaculation. Picture yourself feeling strong, relaxed, and in control of your arousal.

2. Engage All Senses: Make your images as vivid and thorough as possible by engaging all of your senses. Imagine the sights, sounds, smells, and sensations connected with the experience of learning ejaculation control. For example, imagine the sight of your partner's pleasure, the sound of their voice, the scent of your surroundings, and the physical feelings of intimacy.

3. Focus on Positive Emotions: While imagining, focus on feeling positive emotions such as happiness,

confidence, and relationship with your partner. Imagine how it feels to achieve your goals and how it positively impacts your relationship and general well-being.

4. Use Affirmations: Pair your images with positive affirmations or self-talk to support your belief in your ability to achieve ejaculation control. Repeat mantras such as "I am in control of my arousal" or "I can last as long as I want" during your vision practice to improve your attitude and drive.

5. Practice Regularly: Set aside specific time each day to engage in visualization activities. Consistency is key, so make it a daily habit to picture success in learning ejaculation control. Consider adding visualization into your morning or bedtime practice for best success.

6. Stay Flexible: Allow your visualizations to change over time as you move towards your goals. As you experience successes and setbacks, change your visualizations properly to match your present reality and goals. Remain open to new options and opportunities for growth along your trip.

By regularly practicing visualization and immersing yourself in positive mental images of success, you can enhance your drive, resilience, and commitment to learning ejaculation control.

3. Stay Educated:
Continuously seek knowledge and information about ejaculation control techniques, strategies, and tools. Stay updated on latest study results, expert tips, and success stories to inspire and motivate your journey. Explore different methods and adapt them to fit your individual wants and preferences.

Staying informed is crucial for maintaining drive and perseverance in achieving long-term success in learning ejaculation control. Here's how to expand on this strategy:

1. Seek Reliable Sources: Look for reliable sources of information on ejaculation control, such as books, papers, online tools, and professional experts. Choose sources that are evidence-based and grounded in scientific study to ensure you're getting accurate and reliable information.

2. Understand the Physiology: Educate yourself about the bodily and psychological factors that affect ejaculation control. Learn about the processes of arousal, the role of the pelvic floor muscles, and the impact of stress and worry on sexual performance. Understanding these factors can help you build effective methods for handling ejaculation.

3. Explore Techniques: Familiarize yourself with various techniques and methods for better ejaculation control, such as the stop-start method, the squeeze technique, and awareness practices. Experiment with

different methods to discover what works best for you and your partner, and be open to trying new ways as you grow.

4. Stay Updated: Stay abreast of new advances and advancements in the area of sexual health and ejaculation control. Follow respected experts, groups, and sites dedicated to sexual health to stay informed about new study results, innovative treatments, and rising trends in the field.

5. Learn from Others: Seek out personal reports and success stories from individuals who have successfully learned ejaculation control. Hearing about others' experiences and learning from their challenges and successes can provide useful insights and inspiration for your own journey.

6. Educate Your Partner: Involve your partner in your journey towards ejaculation control by educating them about the techniques and tactics you're examining. Open communication and shared understanding can promote support and teamwork, improving your efforts to achieve your goals together.

By staying educated and informed about ejaculation control techniques and strategies, you empower yourself with the information and resources needed to beat obstacles and stay inspired on your journey towards long-term success.

4. Practice Consistently:
Consistency is key to learning ejaculation control.
Incorporate practice lessons into your daily routine,
giving time and effort to improve your skills and
methods. Set aside regular times for practice and
exploration, gradually raising the length and energy
as you progress.

Consistency is important when it comes to learning
ejaculation control. Here's how you can build on this
strategy:

1. Establish a Routine: Integrate practice sessions into
your daily or weekly plan to ensure routine. Choose a
time when you're least likely to be stopped or
distracted, and commit to sticking to your exercise
routine.

2. Start Small: Begin with short practice sessions and
gradually raise the length and intensity over time.
Focus on learning one method or approach at a time
before going on to more advanced practices.

3. Set Realistic Goals: Establish realistic goals for your
practice sessions, taking into account your current
level of skill and experience. Break bigger goals down
into smaller, manageable targets that you can work
towards regularly.

4. Track Your growth: Keep track of your practice
sessions and measure your growth over time. Use a
journal or tracking app to record your efforts, noting

any improvements or hurdles you meet along the way. Celebrate your successes and learn from failures to stay inspired and focused.

5. Stay Committed: Stay committed to your practice habit, even when faced with hurdles or setbacks. Remember that growth takes time and effort, and stay patient and persistent in your goal of success.

6. Be Flexible: Be willing to change your practice schedule as needed based on your changing wants and experiences. Experiment with different methods, approaches, and practice plans to find what works best for you.

By practicing regularly and carefully, you can gradually improve your ejaculation control skills and achieve long-term success in controlling your sexual reaction.

5. Stay Positive:
Maintain a positive mindset and attitude on your journey towards learning ejaculation control. Focus on your strengths, growth, and successes, rather than focusing on mishaps or imagined failures. Embrace a growth attitude that views difficulties as chances for learning and growth, and stay resilient in the face of hurdles.

Maintaining a positive mindset is important for success in learning ejaculation control. Here's how you can build on this strategy:

1. Cultivate Self-Compassion: Be kind and understanding towards yourself, especially during difficult times. Acknowledge that setbacks are a normal part of the learning process and treat yourself with the same kindness you would offer to a friend facing similar challenges.

2. Focus on Progress: Celebrate the progress you make along the way, no matter how small or minor it may seem. Recognize and value the efforts you put into your practice sessions, and accept the changes you experience over time.

3. Reframe Negative Thoughts: Challenge negative thoughts or ideas that may appear during your trip. Instead of viewing losses as failures, reframe them as chances for growth and development. Adopt an upbeat, solution-oriented attitude that focuses on finding helpful ways to overcome challenges.

4. Surround Yourself with Help: Seek help from friends, family members, or a therapist who can give encouragement, direction, and perspective. Share your goals and challenges with trusted individuals who can provide mental support and drive when needed.

5. Practice Gratitude: Cultivate a sense of thanks for the progress you've made, the support you receive, and the chances for growth that come your way. Take time each day to think on the things you're grateful for, no matter how small, and let this happiness fuel your journey towards ejaculation control mastery.

By staying positive and resilient, you can handle the challenges of learning ejaculation control with confidence and drive. Remember that your attitude plays a crucial role in your success, so foster happiness and optimism as you work towards your goals.

6. Celebrate Progress:
Acknowledge and celebrate your progress and successes along the way. Celebrate reaching milestones, overcoming challenges, or adopting winning methods. Reward yourself with small treats or important prizes as a way to reinforce good behavior and motivate continued effort.

Celebrating progress is vital for keeping drive and energy on your journey to learning ejaculation control. Here's how you can successfully execute this strategy:

1. Set Milestones: Break down your bigger goals into smaller, manageable milestones that you can enjoy along the way. These benchmarks could be based on length of control, successful application of techniques, or any other measurable progress indicators.

2. Think on Achievements: Take time to think on your achievements and growth regularly. Acknowledge the efforts you've put in, the improvements you've made, and the difficulties you've solved. This reflection helps

reinforce a sense of success and keeps you inspired to continue going forward.

3. Reward Yourself: Treat yourself to prizes or incentives whenever you hit a milestone or make a major breakthrough. These rewards could be anything that brings you joy, such as indulging in your favorite meal, getting yourself a small gift, or having a relaxing activity. The key is to choose rewards that are important to you and strengthen your commitment to your goals.

4. Share Your Success: Share your wins with encouraging friends, family members, or a trusted confidant. Celebrating your success with others not only improves the joy of accomplishment but also strengthens your support network and reinforces your commitment to your goals.

5. Keep a Progress book: Maintain a book or log where you record your progress, goals, and wins. Reflecting on how far you've come can be incredibly motivating and inspiring, especially during times when you may feel defeated or facing difficulties.

6. Stay Positive: Cultivate a positive approach towards your growth and successes. Focus on the effort you've put in and the changes you've made, rather than dwelling on any setbacks or flaws. Remember that growth is a journey, and every step forward is worth celebrating.

By celebrating your progress along the way, you'll
stay driven, inspired, and committed to learning
ejaculation control. Embrace each success as a proof
to your dedication and resilience, and let it fuel your
continued efforts towards your goals.

7. Seek Support:
Surround yourself with a helpful network of friends,
family, or peers who understand and encourage your
goals. Share your experiences, challenges, and
achievements with others who can offer empathy,
encouragement, and useful advice. Consider joining
support groups or online communities dedicated to
ejaculation control to meet with like-minded people
and gain useful insights and inspiration.

Seeking help from others can be a powerful tool in
your journey to learning ejaculation control. Here's
how you can successfully leverage support:

1. Build an accepting Network: Surround yourself with
friends, family members, or peers who are
understanding, non-judgmental, and accepting of
your goals. Share your goals and difficulties with
individuals who can offer understanding,
encouragement, and useful advice.

2. Join Support Groups: Consider joining support
groups or online communities dedicated to ejaculation
control and sexual health. These groups provide a
safe and supportive setting where you can connect

with others having similar challenges, share experiences, and swap tips and strategies for success.

3. Attend Therapy or Counseling: Seeking professional help from a therapist or counselor skilled in sexual health problems can provide useful advice and support. A trained therapist can help you explore underlying factors adding to ejaculation control issues, develop coping strategies, and provide personalized advice tailored to your unique needs.

4. Engage in Open conversation: Foster open and honest conversation with your partner about your goals, challenges, and wishes related to ejaculation management. Sharing your journey with your partner can improve your relationship, enhance intimacy, and create a supportive environment where you can work together towards shared happiness and joy.

5. Educate Yourself: Take the initiative to educate yourself about ejaculation control techniques, tactics, and tools. Stay informed about latest study findings, expert advice, and available treatment choices. Knowledge enables you to make informed choices, fight for yourself, and actively join in your own journey towards mastery.

6. Be Selective with Support: Choose your support network wisely and seek advice from individuals who show understanding, kindness, and respect for your goals. Avoid negative forces or individuals who undermine your efforts or stop you from following

your goals. Surround yourself with happiness and support to stay inspired and focused on your road to success.

By getting help from a supportive network, you can gain useful insights, encouragement, and practical advice to beat obstacles and achieve your goals in mastering ejaculation control. Remember that you're not alone in your journey, and calling out for help is a sign of power and resilience.

8. Stay Flexible:
Be open to adapting and adjusting your method as needed based on comments, experiences, and changing circumstances. Stay flexible and ready to try with different techniques, strategies, and approaches to find what works best for you. Embrace an attitude of ongoing growth and polishing as you work towards long-term success in learning ejaculation control.

Staying open is crucial in your road to learning ejaculation control. Here's how you can retain flexibility:

1. Adapt to Feedback: Be open to feedback from yourself, your partner, or trusted people in your support network. Pay attention to what works well and what doesn't, and be ready to adjust your method properly.

2. Experiment with Different Techniques: Don't be afraid to try out new techniques, strategies, or tasks

to see what works best with you. Keep an open mind and be ready to step outside your comfort zone to discover new possibilities.

3. Listen to Your Body: Tune into your body's signs and cues during sexual action. Notice how different techniques or methods impact your excitement levels and ejaculation control, and change your actions accordingly.

4. Be Patient and Persistent: Mastery takes time and effort, so be patient with yourself as you handle obstacles and failures along the way. Stay committed to your goals and keep going forward, even if success seems slow at times.

5. Embrace Trial and Error: Recognize that finding the right method to ejaculation control may involve some trial and error. Don't get frustrated by failures or initial difficulties; instead, view them as useful learning experiences that add to your growth and development.

6. Seek Professional Advice: If you're fighting to make progress on your own, don't hesitate to seek advice from a skilled therapist, counselor, or healthcare provider focusing on sexual health. They can offer personalized help, tools, and resources to support you on your trip.

7. Stay Open to Change: Be ready to change and evolve your method over time as you gain new

insights and experiences. What works for you today may not necessarily work tomorrow, so stay flexible and responsive to changing conditions.

By staying flexible and adaptable, you can overcome hurdles more effectively and increase your chances of long-term success in learning ejaculation control. Remember that flexibility is a key trait of resilience and growth, so accept it as you work towards your goals.

# Conclusion

In conclusion, "Ejaculation Mastery: 10 Easy-to-Follow Strategies for Delaying Climax and Lasting Longer in Bed" has provided you with useful tools and techniques to take control of your sexual experiences. Throughout this journey, we've studied various strategies, from sensory control and breathing techniques to mindfulness and conversation, all aimed at helping you prolong pleasure and improve closeness.

As you think about the key points covered in this book, remember that lasting longer in bed is not just about physical techniques but also about attitude, communication, and general well-being. By applying these strategies regularly and with commitment, you can develop a fulfilling sex life characterized by greater confidence, intimacy, and happiness.

I encourage you to take what you've learned and apply it in your own sexual adventures. Be patient with yourself as you handle hurdles and failures, and enjoy your progress along the way. Remember that mastery is a path, not a location, and each step you take brings you closer to achieving your goals.

Above all, value open conversation with your partner, as their support and understanding are invaluable on this trip. Together, you can discover new areas of pleasure, strengthen your connection, and create unique moments that enrich your relationship.

With drive, practice, and a positive mindset, you have the power to unlock your full potential in the bedroom and experience the joys of ejaculation control. Here's to a fulfilling and satisfying sex life filled with happiness, intimacy, and permanent satisfaction.

Here's a review of the key points and techniques for delaying climax and staying longer in bed:

1. Sensory Control: Experiment with different amounts of touch, pressure, and excitement to find what works best for you. Slow down or stop when nearing climax to allow desire to plateau.

2. Breathing Techniques: Practice deep, slow breathing to calm the nervous system and control desire. Sync your breath with your moves to keep control and prolong pleasure.

3. Mindfulness and Distraction: Stay present in the moment and prevent your mind from moving to thoughts of climax. Engage in light distraction or mindfulness methods to change attention away from arousal.

4. Change of Pace and Position: Vary the pace and rhythm of closeness to lengthen the experience. Experiment with different sexual positions that offer less pleasure or allow for greater control over desire.

5. Pelvic Floor Exercises: Strengthen these muscles through kegel exercises to improve ejaculatory control. Practice tightening and calming these muscles during contact to delay ejaculation.

6. Conversation and Partner Collaboration: Open and honest conversation about wants, tastes, and goals can help both partners work together to control arousal and increase joy.

7. Sensate Focus: Take turns touching and exploring each other's bodies, focused on pleasure and connection rather than reaching release. This builds closeness and prolongs pleasure.

8. Visualization and Mental Imagery: Use visualization methods to picture yourself in a calm and relaxed state, free from performance pressure or worry. Picture yourself lasting longer and loving the trip of intimacy with your mate.

9. Scheduled Ejaculation: Incorporate scheduled ejaculation sessions into your sexual practice to gradually build up energy and control over time.

10. Self-awareness and Reflection: Reflect on sexual experiences, spot trends or causes leading to premature ejaculation, and track success of different tactics to tailor your approach.

These tactics, when practiced regularly and with patience, can help you delay climax and extend the length of intercourse, leading to a more enjoyable and fulfilling sex life.

Dear readers,

As you start on your journey to learn ejaculation control and enhance your sexual experience, remember that change takes time and patience. Each of the methods described in this book takes practice and dedication, but the rewards are well worth the effort.

By applying these strategies into your life, you're not only investing in your sexual health and happiness but also strengthening the relationship with your partner. Communication, experimentation, and mutual discovery are key components of a happy sex life.

Don't be frustrated by failures or challenges along the way. Instead, view them as chances for growth and learning. Stay committed to your goals, stay open to new situations, and stay connected with your partner.

Remember, you have the power to shape your sexual experience and create a satisfying sex life. With determination, perseverance, and the methods described in this book, you can achieve greater happiness, intimacy, and pleasure in your interactions.

Here's to your journey towards ejaculation mastery
and a lifetime of satisfying sexual adventures.

Best thoughts,


Patti W. Nieves

www.ingramcontent.com/pod-product-compliance
Lightning Source LLC
Chambersburg PA
CBHW050806260726
48660CB00004B/1286